The A to Z of
Reproductive & Sexual Organs

Introduction

Because of space limitations it was not possible to include the organs of reproduction, in the book **the A to Z of Major Organs**; hence this book was needed to fill that gap. Hopefully it has done the job. Where possible, comparisons are made between the female & male. There are also structural considerations of sexuality. I continue to receive suggestions and feedback in reference to these books and I cannot stress how valuable these are to me. I feel with each book a new level is reached and this is due to constant vigilance. You, who write to me, shape the order of future ti̶̶̶̶̶̶̶̶̶ nge the format of the books, so please keep thi̶ ill form another valuable chapter in begets structure beget Human mechanics is a

The A to Zs may be view **www.amandasatoz.co** **http://www.aspcnphar** Feedback may be left at **anatomy.update@gmail.** ......icalamanda@gmail.com and it is always appreciated.

Acknowledgement

Thank you Aspen Pharmacare Australia for your support and assistance in this valuable project, particularly Mr. Greg Lan, Rob Koster, Richard Clement and Peter Penn.

Dedication

To my A to Z -" Hello Ali & Zoe!" Quentin & Jody and Colin, who has been very supportive of this project, listened to my ideas with patience and at times great fortitude.

How to use this book

The format of this A to Z book has been maintained. The common terms section enlarged & illustrated. So as usual think of it and then find it is the motto of the A to Zs and continues to be the structure behind the books.

Thank you
A. L. Neill
BSc MSc MBBS PhD FACBS

ISBN 978-1-921930-04-1

1

TABLE OF CONTENTS

Abbreviations, Acronyms & Symbols

Note these abbreviations include those in common use in the study and examination of reproductive organs as well as the ones used in this book.

A

a	= artery
aa	= anastomosis (ses)
AA	= amino acid
Ab	= antibody
ACTH	= adrenocorticotropic hormone / adrenal cortical hormone
ADH	= antidiuretic hormone
adj.	= adjective
ADP	= adenosine diphosphate
Ag	= antigen
aka	= also known as
alt.	= alternative
AMP	= adenosine monophosphate
ANS	= autonomic nervous system
ant.	= anterior
AS	= Alternative Spelling, generally referring to the diff. b/n British & American spelling
ATP	= adenosine triphosphate

B

B	= blood
b	= bone
bb	= basal bodies
bc	= because
BDSM	= bondage discipline / sadomasochism
BE	= breast examination

B M

BM	= basement membrane / basal lamina / terminal lamina / plasma lamina
b/n	= between
br	= branch
BS	= Blood Supply
BvB	= Balbiani's vitelline body

C

CC	= cerebral cortex
c.f.	= compared to
CL	= corpus luteum
CM	= cellular membrane / plasma membrane
CNS	= central nervous system
Co	= coccygeal
COC	= combined oral contraceptives
CP	= cervical plexus
collat.	= collateral
Cr	= cranial
CT	= connective tissue

D

DNA	= deoxyribonucleic acid
DOPA	= dihydroxyphenylalanine
DT	= digestive tract
diff.	= difference(s)
dist.	= distal
DM	= dura mater
DT	= digestive tract

E

E	= energy
e.g.	= example
EAM	= external acoustic meatus
EAS	= external anal sphincter
ec	= extracellular (outside the cell)
ER	= endoplasmic reticulum
ext.	= extensor (as in muscle to extend across a joint)
Ex	= examination

F

FAS	= foetal alcohol syndrome
FB	= foreign body
FHR	= foetal heart rate
FSH	= follicle stimulating hormone

G

GA	= Golgi apparatus
GALT	= gut associated lymphoid tissue
GB	= gall bladder
GDM	= gestational diabetes mellitus
GH	= growth hormone
gld	= gland
GIT	= gastro-intestinal tract
Gk.	= Greek
GM	= grey matter
GN	= Golgi network

H

H	= hormone
H&E	= haematoxylin & eosin
HIV	= human immunodeficiency virus
HP	= high pressure
HPV	= human papilloma virus
HR	= heart rate
HRT	= hormone replacement therapy
HT	= hormone therapy

I

IAM	= internal acoustic meatus
IAS	= internal anal sphincter
IBS	= irritable bowel syndrome
ic	= intracellular (inside the cell)
If	= inflammation
In	= infection
IUCD	= intrauterine contraceptive device
IVF	= in vitro fertilization

J

Jc	= junctional complex
jt(s)	= joints = articulations

K

L

l	= lymphatic
L	= lumbar / left
LH	= luteinizing hormone
LI	= large intestine
lig	= ligament
LM	= labia majora
LMi	= labia minora
LMP	= last menstrual period
LP	= lamina propria
LT	= lymphoid tissue
Lt.	= Latin
LIF	= left iliac fossa
LUQ	= left upper quadrant

© A. L. Neill

M

m = muscle
med. = medial
mem = membrane
mito = mitochondrion (a)
mm = mucous membrane
mRNA = messenger RNA
MTP = medical termination of pregnancy
mv = microvillus (i)

N

N (s) = nerve(s)
NAD = normal (size, shape)
NAD = no abnormality detected
NB = newborn
NM = nuclear membrane / nucleolemma
NR = nerve root origin
NS = nerve supply / nervous system
NT = nervous tissue
nv = neurovascular bundle

O

0 = origin
OC = Oral Contraceptives

P

PB = perineal body
PID = pelvic inflammatory disease
pl. = plural
ParaNS = parasympathetic nervous system
PDA = patent ductus arteriosis
PID = pelvic inflammatory disease

PN = peripheral nerve
post. = posterior
proc. = process
prox. = proximal
PS = pubic symphysis
PV = penis vagina

R

R = right / resistance
RIF = right iliac fossa
RNA = ribonucleic acid
RR = respiratory rate
rRNA = ribosomal RNA
RUQ = right upper quadrant

S

SA = sexual activity
SAB = spontaneous abortion
SB = spina bifida
SBE = self breast examination
SC = spinal cord
SE = side effects
SI = small intestine
sing. = singular
SM = sadomasochistic
SN = spinal nerve
SP = sacral plexus
SS = signs and symptoms
STD = sexually transmitted diseases
subcut. = subcutaneous (just under the skin)
supf = superficial
SymNS = sympathetic nervous system

T

T	= thoracic / tissue
T_3	= tri-iodothyronine
T_4	= thyroxine
TNF	= tumour necrosis factor
tRNA	= transfer RNA / transport RNA
TSH	= thyroid stimulating hormone / thyrotropic H / thyrotrophic H
tw	= terminal web

U

UG	= urogenital
US	= ultrasound
UTI	= urinary tract infection
UVJ	= uterovesicular junction

V

V	= vein
v	= very
VD	= vas deferens

W

WM	= white matter
w/n	= within
w/o	= without
wrt	= with respect to

X

YZ

ZA	= zonula adherens
ZO	= zonula occludens / tight junction
ZP	= zona pellucida

Symbols

&	= and
∩	= intersection with

Pronunciation Key & Colour Guide

Most terms are listed in black

Pathological terms are in green

Prefixes and Suffixes are in blue

Specific sexual meanings of terms are listed separately in maroon

The pronunciation guide to words in this section are in bold red lettering

Stressed syllables are in **CAPITAL LETTERS**

Vowel sounds are pronounced as indicated below

A	May	ay
	map	a
	mark	ah
E	Me	ee
	met	ə
	term	ur
I	eye / sight	ï
	tin	i
O	go	oh
	mother	uh
	mop	o
	more	or
	boy	oi
	lose	oo
	nook	oe
	loose	ou
U	blue	ou
	cute	ew
	cut	uh
Y	family	ee
	myth	i
	eye	ï

Common Terms used to describe the eyes; their structure & functions

A

a- without, lack of, no

ab- away from, negative

Abdomen *Lt. abdomen = the belly,* the part of the trunk b/n thorax & the perineum,

Abduction: *Lt. ab = from, & ductum =* led, hence, movement from; verb - abduct. (≠ adduction)

Abduction AKA Captivation / Kidnapping to carry a person away by force used in SA; a minor form is the custom of carrying the bride across the threshold indicating a "carrying off" of the bride

Aberrant *Lt. ab = from, & errare =* to wander, hence, deviating from normal.

Abrasion (ab-RAY-shon) - removal of the surface layer(s) of the skin due to trauma, if full thickness it exposes the dermis underneath & the leaves the surface susceptible to In.

Absorption (ab-SORB-shun) the passage of material, such as an embryo, from a lumen of an organ into another body space, T or cell

ac- toward, near to, addition to

Abstinence AKA Aphallatia AKA Celibacy refraining from SA - may be defined in various ways the commonest being the abstinence from coitus.

Accessory *Lt. accessum = added,* hence, supplementary.

Achalasia (AY-kal-ay-si-ya) failure of relaxation of smooth muscle

Acini (AS-i-nee) clusters of cells which face a lumen and are often part of an exocrine gland that secrete digestive enzymes. *sing. acinus (AS-in-us) adj. acinar*

Acmegenesis AKA Orgasm

Acne (AK-nee) *Gk: acme = point or achne = to chaff* an inflammatory condition of the pilosebacious unit – hair unit in the skin - exacerbated by progesterone in the female & reduced by oestrogen

Acomoclitic preference for hairless genitals

acou- to hear, pertaining to hearing

acoustic- (ah-KOOS-tik) *adj.Gk. akoustikos = hearing* related to hearing; pertaining to hearing & sounds

Acoustophilia arousal by sounds. This may be musical &/or vocalizations of the person or the partner.

acro- extremity

Acrophilia arousal from heights

Acrotomorphilia arousal for amputees

Actin (AK-tin) *Gk: actinos – ray* the contractile protein that makes up the major portion of thin filaments in muscle fibers.

Actirasty exposure by the sun causing arousal

acu- sudden, sharp , severe

Acucullophallia AKA Circumcision

Acute (AK-yewt) – *Gk: acu- acus = needle* sharp, sudden onset + short course pathological process – used to describe any condition which starts suddenly & is of short duration; may be associated with a sharp needle-like pain of relatively short duration ≠ chronic, although 2 separate processes they may co-exist.

ad- near, toward

Additus *Lt. = entrance, opening*

Adduction: *Lt. ad = to*, & *ductum = led*, hence, movement towards; *verb - adduct.* (≠ abduction)

aden- gland

Adenoid: *Gk. aden = a gland, eidos = shape or form.*

Adenohypophysis AKA the Anterior Lobe of the Pituitary Gland. It is composed of glandular epithelium. The adenohypophysis secretes numerous Hs, several of which affect the activity of other endocrine glands, including the reproductive organs/glands.

Adenomyosis presence of glandular tissue on the myometrium generally from the endometrium *see also Endometriosis*

Adhesion: *Lt. ad = to*, & *haesus = stuck*

Adipose (AD-i-pohs) *Lt. adeps = fat, hence fatty* a CT whose cells (adipocytes) are highly specialized for lipid storage.

Adjuvant *Lt auivare = to aid*, hence a pharmacological or other agent which aids the primary Tx c.f. adjuvant therapy or immunological adjuvants which stimulate the immune response

Adnexa (AD-nex-uh) appendices or adjunct parts e.g.: in the uterus, the supportive ligaments & ovaries & in the skin, the hair & nails: additional structures pertaining to the main structure; extras *adj. adnexal; pl adnexae*

Adrenal: *Lt. ad = towards, at, ren = kidney*, situated near the kidney (AKA suprarenal) *adj. adrenergic Gk. ergon = work*, stimuli which cause the adrenal (suprarenal) gland to produce adrenaline; also indicates neurons or pathways which use adrenaline as a transmitter.

Adrenocorticotropic hormone AKA Corticotropic H AKA Adrenotropic H a hormone which causes the adrenal cortex to grow and secrete more Hs

Adultery SA outside marriage, including coitus.

Adventitia (ad-ven-TISH-yah) the outermost covering of an organ or tissue *(see also Serosa, Tunica Externa)*.

aero- air, pertaining to gas

af- near, toward, addition to

Agenobiosis marriage relationship w/o SA

agglut- **(a-GLOOT)** to glue

aggreg- to crowd together, to flock

Agonist: *Gk. agonistes = rival*, hence, a muscle in apparent contest with another, (a prime mover).

Agorophilia arousal from open spaces

Agrexorphilia arousal from the knowledge that someone else is aware of the SA

Ala (AY-lar) *Lt. wing, hence a wing-like process; pl. alae (AY-lee)* referring to the wing or flattened part of a bone particularly if there are other shapes in the bone which are not wide & flat as in the Inominate / hip.

alb- white

Alba: *Lt. albus = white*

Albicans: *Lt. = becoming white*

Albuginea: *Lt. albus = white, Gk. gen = form*, like boiled white of an egg.

Alberran's gland - the portion of the median lobe of the prostate immediately underlying the uvula of the urinary bladder

-algia *Gk: algos = pain* **(AL-jee-uh)** -

Algolagnia *Gk: algos = pain & lagnia = lust* arousal from pain when engaging in SA

Alimentary: *adj. Lt. alimentum = food*, e.g., alimentary canal.

alipo- pertaining to fat

Allantois: *Gk. allantos = sausage, eidos = like*, form.

allo- other, different, abnormal

Alloerasty arousal by nudity

Allopellia form of Voyeurism, where the couple being watched are engaged in coitus

Allorgasmia arousal from visualizing another person than the partner in SA

Alopecia (AL-oh –peesh-uh) *Gk alopekia =fox mange* hence baldness, loss of hair

Alphamegamia arousal b/n partners from significantly different age groups

Altocalciphilia arousal by high heels, generally pointed stiletto heels; high heel fetish

Alveolus: *Lt. = a basin*, hence any small air filled hollow or cavity. *pl. - alveoli, adj.- alveolar*, after holes in a tissue

Amatripsis masturbation by rubbing labia together *see also Masturbation*

ambi- both, about, around

Ambi-sexual AKA Androgynophilia AKA Bisexual

Amenorrhoea (AY-men-or-REE-ah) absence of menstral bleeding in a premenopausal female > 3 months

Amastia absence of all or part of the breast tissue &/or its components, this may be iatrogenic or congenital

amin(o)- an organic substance containing nitrogen

Amnion *Gk: amnios = bowl* **(AM-nee-yoh)** – membranes surrounding the foetus

Amniocentesis sampling of the amniotic fluid generally with a view to diagnosing genetic disease in the developing foetus, must be performed > 3mnths pregnancy, so that there is sufficient fluid to sample; has a risk of damaging the pregnancy

Amniotomy AKA surgically induced labour

Amomaxia coitus in a parked car

Ampulla: *Lt. = a two-handed flask*, a local dilatation of a tube. c.f. the oviducts

Amychesis scratching during SA

an- without, lack of, not

an(a)- up, back, again, excessive

Anaemia AS Anemia *w/o blood* hence lack of RBCs

Anal sex SA involving the anus - note there are a number of terms to describe various forms of this SA, some of which are included in this text. Those included are the commonest used in medical terminology, but do not include the many slang terms used which are often confined to local use.

Androgen AKA Androgenic H AKA Testoid the broad term for any natural or synthetic compound, that stimulates or controls the development & maintenance of male sexual characteristics e.g. testosterone, dihydrotestosterone (DHT) which is responsible for the development of the scrotum & testis & later prostate growth & male pattern baldness.

Andropause male equivalent of menopause with ↓ testosterone

Androsodomy anal sex with a male partner

Anemia AS Anaemia a deficiency in the number &/or quality of RBCs

Anilingus AKA Rimming oral sex in & around the anus

angio- (ANJ-ee-oh) to do with BVs

Anions negatively charged atoms or radicals e.g. Cl-, OH-

Annulus fibrosis the peripheral fibrous ring around the intervertebral disc

anomalo- uneven, irregular

Anomeatia anal sex with a female partner

Anovulation lack of ovulation

Anorgasmia inability to reach an orgasm – generally wrt women

Apareunia absence or inability to have sexual intercourse

ante- (AN-tee) before

Antenatal *Lt. ante = before, & nato = birth* hence before the birth

antero- anterior, forward

Anteflexion: *Lt. ante = before, & flexere = to bend*, ant. angulation b/n the body & cervix of the uterus

Anteversion: *Lt. ante = before, & versum = turned*, hence, the ant. angulation b/n cervix uterus & the vagina

anti- against, combating

Antibody / Antigen, proteins involved in the immune system – antibodies *Abs* are produced by the body in reaction to antigens *Ags* proteins or materials found on the surface of FBs introduced to the body forming the *Ab/Ag* complex.
AutoAbs are those Abs which develop against the *Ags* of the host - i.e. autoimmune e.g. after a vasectomy the body may develop *AutoAbs* against sperm

Antrum: *Gk. antron - cave*, hence a space in a bone or organ.

Apocrine secretions which take off the cytoplasm of the apex of the cell as well e.g. in breast lactating gland cells

ap- toward , near to

ap- away from derived from, separation

Aperture (AP-ert-yew-er) an opening or space b/n bones or w/n a bone.

Apex (AY-pex) the extremity of a conical or pyramidal structure. The apex of the heart is the rounded, inferior tip that points to the L side.

Aphrodisiac (AF-roh-diz-ee-ak) substances which enhance sexual arousal

Apistia AKA Adultery

Apoptysis (AP-pop-te-sis) *Gk aptos = to drop out* describes pockets of dead or dying cells - found in all organs wedged b/n healthy cells so it is thought to be a physiological phenomenon of normal aging or cellular weeding out e.g. in the liver, ovary

Appendicular refers to the appendices of the axial i.e. in the skeleton, the arms & legs which hang from the axial skeleton; this also includes the pectoral & pelvic girdles *noun appendix* as in the vermiform appendix

Arbor *Gk treelike branches – arborizing*, branching

arch- chief, first, beginning

Areata/areatus (a-REE-ar-tar) *Lt circumscribed areas*, c.f. alopecia areata – specific areas of hairlessness - baldness

Areola (ar-EE-oh-lar) *Lt. small, open space* hence small, open spaces as in the areolar part of the breast which open onto the surface and allow lactation adj. areolar used to describe a type of CT with sparse protein fibres in the matrix.

Arsometry AKA Anal Sex

Asceticism religious self denial often includes celibacy

Asherman's syndrome AKA intra-uterine adhesions

Asphyxiaphilia arousal from lack of oxygen, has resulted in deaths when done in a solo situation as there is no-one to reverse the oxygen deprivation once the subject is in a coma *see Auto erotic asphyxia*

asthen- weak, weakness

Artificial insemination depositing of sperm into the vagina using a vehicle other than the penis, generally with a view to causing conception

Astyphia AKA Impotence

Asynodia celibacy due to impotence

Atelectasis (AT-e-lek-TAY-sis) *Gk ateles- incomplete , ektasis* – opening hence incomplete opening of the lungs, generally in premature infants

Atopy (AY-top-ee) *Gk atopis = out of place* group of diseases characterized by the tendency to have a severe hypersensitive reaction to common materials as in the RT, GIT & skin adj. atopy = allergic as in atopic dermatitis = skin If

Atresia (A-treez-ee-uh): *Gk. a = negative, & tresis = a hole*, an absence or closure of a body orifice or tubular organ, generally by fibrous scarring

atreto (a-TREE-toh)- closed, imperforate

Atrium (AY-tree-um) *Lt. = entrance hall, adj.- atrial* referring to any chambers which lie before a major chamber as in the heart *pl. - atria.*

Atrophy (a-TROH-fee) *Gk. a = negative, & trophe = food* wasting away deterioration of a T or organ from lack of use or food

Atypical (AY-tip-i-kal) not usual – often used to describe possible cancerous cells or tissue

Augmentation enhancement c.f. breast implants augment the shape of the breast by 1-2 cup sizes usually any more than this and the shape and integrity of the breast & its support structures may be compromised *see also Implants*

Autagonistophilia AKA Exhibitionism

auto- (OR-toh) self, spontaneous

Auto erotic asphyxia sexual stimulation caused by deprivation of oxygen in a solo situation. This activity has a real risk of harm or death to the subject, if the person lapses into a coma.

Autocrine secretions of the cell influence other like cells & its own function

Autolysis (OR-tol-e-sis) *Gk auto = self , lysis = dissolving* - hence the process of self destruction of a cell or tissue

aux- (ORKS) help, growth, increase

Axilla *Lt. axilla = armpit* pertaining to the triangular region at the top of the UL & the upper thoracic wall – *the underarm*

Axis (AX-is) *Lt. axis = the central line of a body or part thereof, especially the imaginary line around which rotation takes place* refers to the head and trunk (vertebrae, ribs and sternum) of the body. *adj. axial (AX-see-al) pl. axes*

Azoospermia AKA no sperm count small but not measurable sperm may be present; however this result indicates a low fertility

B

Balanitis *Gk balano = penis* If of the glans penis, resulting in an inflammatory ooze & constriction of the foreskin *see also Phimosis*

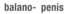

balano- penis

Balanoposthitis AKA Balanitis

Balbiani body a transient collection of organelles, inclusions & molecules that assembles adjacent to the nucleus of the oöcytes.

Baldness *see Alopecia*

Ball's valves AKA anal valves.

Bandl's ring the diagonal retraction band (2) of the uterine muscle wall which results from continued uterine contraction present in obstructed labours of the 2nd or later pregnancies. Progressive contraction leads to a thinning & separation of the lower (1t) segment & thickened contracted upper third (1c) which if unchecked leads to uterine rupture (3), & non delivery of the baby(4). The resulting engorgement in the vagina

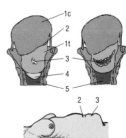

© A. L. Neill

(4) & elsewhere leads to dehydration. Examination of the supine woman can discern the banding in the abdomen, softening below & hard T above.

bar- pressure

Barbae *Gk = beard*

Bartholin's glands AKA Greater Vestibular Glands

bary- low, heavy, deep difficult

Basement membrane (BM) a thin layer of extracellular material & CT stroma that underlies every epithelium.

basi- foundation, base

baso- base c.f. acid / base & in the bottom — the basal layer

Bell's muscle the muscular strands from the ureteric orifices to the uvula, bounding the trigone of the urinary bladder

Benign (BEE-nïn), *Fr benignus = kind* hence not harmful or dangerous, ≠ malignant, indicating a mild disease or a mild non-malignant cancer

bi- twice , two, double

Bifid: *adj. Lt. bis = double, & findo = to split.*

Bifurcate: *Lt. bis = double, & furco = fork,* hence to divide into two.

Bilateral: *Lt. bi = two, lateral = side,* hence, pertaining to two (both) sides.

bin- twice , two, double

bio- (bï-oh) life

Biopsy (Bï-op-see) a piece of T removed for microscopic examination — usually from a live person e.g. cervical biopsy - a punch of tissue is taken or in cases of invasive cells - a cone biopsy - shown below, which is then cut up & examined histologically

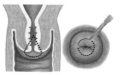

Bisexuality attraction to both sexes

blast- undifferentiated immature

Blastocyst a group of cells derived from the fertilized ovum, which have not yet differentiated, but has formed a central fluid filled area

Blastocyte a single cell in the blastocyst / blastoma

Blastoma a solid core of cell from the fertilized ovum

Blowjob AKA oral penile sex referring to the mouth penile sexual contact performed in various ways & positions but having in common the fact of sexual arousal via oral contact

Bondage binding in the pursuit of SA, often part of SM rituals

brachy- (brak-EE) short

brady- slow

Bradycupia slow movement in SA partic. penetration

Branchia (BRANK-ee-uh): *Gk. = gills, adj.- branchial.*

Breast crease the line formed when the breast folds over the chest - viewed by raising the breast & viewing the "crease" visible across the chest - should curve upwards with the curve of the breast tissue but may be horizontal in small high-waisted women or overweight women associated with an increased area of fat in the axillary region

Break-through -bleeding bleeding in the middle of the menstral cycle which indicate irregular H levels - if the person is on OCs it indicates a need for adjustment of these Hs - generally a reduction in the progesterone levels &/or ↑ oestrogen levels

brevi- short

Brevis: *Lt. = short* - c.f. brief.

Brunn's cell nests epithelial cell masses in the male urethra.

Buck's fascia AKA deep fascia of the penis

Buggery AKA Anal sex

Bulimia (BULL-ee-mee-ya) *Lt bous = ox + limos = hunger* hence huge episodic binging of food eating followed by self induced vomiting or excessive exercising, associated with eating disorders prevalent among young women & assoc with amenorrhea if severe

Bulla: *Lt. = bubble.* pl bullae

Burns' ligament falciform margin of the fascia lata at the saphenous opening

Bursa (BER-suh) *Gk. = a purse*, hence a flattened sac containing a film of fluid, formed from friction b/n tissue layers, generally skin, to alleviate tissue trauma. *pl bursae*

C

cac- (KAK) bad, diseased, deformed , ill

caen-(SEEN) new, recent

Camper's fascia superficial layer of the subcutaneous tissue (superficial fascia) of the abdomen.

Canal: *Lt. canalis = a water-pipe or canal. adj canular* (canicule - small canal)

Canal of Nuck AKA patent processus vaginalis peritonei in the female

Canaliculus (kan-al-LIK-yew-lus) a small channel *pl. canaliculi.* diminutive of canal.

Cancellous: *adj. Lt. cancelli = grating or lattice.*

Cancer (KAN-ser): *Lt crab* - describing originally the crab-like invasion of cancer cells spreading out into normal tissue – malignant neoplasms

Cannula AS Canula (KAN-yew-lar) *Lt cannula = little roof / a tube* hence a tube which is inserted into the body

Capacitation maintenance of the internal environment of the oviduct to facilitate penetration of the spermatozoa into the ovum

Capillary (kap-IL-lar-ee) *Lt. capillaris = hair-like*, hence a very thin BV that interconnects arterioles with venules. The capillary wall is a single cell layer in thickness, & is the only site of nutrient diffusion b/n the BS & body cells.

Capsule (KAPS-yew-l) *Lt. capsa = box*, hence an enclosing membrane

Caput: *Lt. = head., adj.- capitate = having a head* (c.f. decapitate).

Caput medusae: *Lt. caput = head, Gk. = Medusa* a mythical female with ugly & with snake like hair.

Carcinogen (KAR-sin-oh-jen) material which leads to cancer formation

Carcinoma (KAR-sin-oh-mah) a malignant growth originating from epithelial cells

Carcinoma – *in situ* pre-invasive cancer still lying in the confines of normal tissue not having broken through the BM but with neoplastic changes, e.g. in the cervix

Cardinal: *Lt. cardinalis = principal*, honce something of primary importance.

Castration (CAS-tray-shon) removal of the genitalia generally in ref. to the male - note if the prostate gland remains it is still possible to have an orgasm. In the female castration is the removal of the ovaries, which does not interfere with the ability to orgasm. Casterati - young boys castrated to preserve their voice & maintain their physique.

Catamenia (KAT-uh-meen-ee-yuh) AKA Menses AKA Menstruation *Gk Katamenios = monthly*

Catheter (KATH-e-ter) a tube which is forced through an orifice to allow for passage which has been obstructed e.g. if the bladder is obstructed it is catheterized forcing open the urethra which may be being closed by external pressure from an hypertrophied prostate

Cauda: *Lt. = tail, adj.- caudate - having a tail.*

Cauda equina: *Lt. = a horse's tail.* adj caudal hence toward the tail, inferior (in human anatomy), note legs are inferior not caudal

Cava: *Lt. cavum = cave, hollow adj cavernous containing caverns or cave-like spaces.*

Cave of Retzius AKA retropubic space AKA prevesical space

Cavity: (KAV-it-ee) *Lt. cavitas = a hollow* hence an open area or sinus w/n a bone or formed by 2 or more bones. (in dentistry a pathological hollow in the bone – tooth).

Celibacy Abstinence of sex

Cell (SELL) the basic living unit of multi-cellular organisms.

Cell body the portion of a neuron containing the nucleus & much of the cytoplasm. **(AKA the SOMA).**

Celom AS Coelom

cen- general, common - new recent

centi- hundredth part, hundred

Centriole (SEN-tree-ohl) cylindrical structures w/n the cytoplasm of a cell, consisting of microtubules, which play a role in cell division.

cephal- head

Cephalic (KEF–al-ik) *Gk. kephale = head* pertaining to the head

Cephalhaematoma haemorrhage in the skull of the NB, blood b/n the skull & periosteum

cer- (ser) wax

cerat- (kerat) cornea / horny tissue

Cerclage stitch or ring in the cervix (1) to prevent miscarriage due to an incompetent cervix (B) ensuring the os is closed (A)

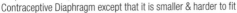
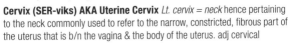

Cervical cap a rubber cap which fits over the cervix and prevents the passage of sperm when in place; similar to a Contraceptive Diaphragm except that it is smaller & harder to fit

Cervix (SER-viks) AKA Uterine Cervix *Lt. cervix = neck* hence pertaining to the neck commonly used to refer to the narrow, constricted, fibrous part of the uterus that is b/n the vagina & the body of the uterus. adj cervical

Cervix Uteri the thinning elongation, softening & effacement of the cervix in pregnancy where the cervix is incorporated in to the lower third of the uterus

cheil- lip (cheel-)

chemo- relating to chemistry, chemically induced (keem-oh)

Chemotaxis (KEEM-oh-tax-is) cellular phenomenon of moving towards or away from specific areas due to the chemical present

chiro- hand (kyro-)

Chloasma (KLOH-az-muh) AKA Melasma hyperpigmentation of the sensitive areas of the skin exposed to sunlight due to H imbalance, or pregnancy, even if corrected it may take 9 mnths for the skin to return to its original colour

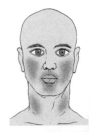

Chorda: *Lt. = cord.*

chori- (kor-ee-) protective membrane

Choroid (KO-royd) part of the vascular tunic covering of the eyeball. It lines most of the internal surface of the sclera, forming the middle layer of the wall of the eye.

Chorion (KAW-ree-on): *Gk chorios = membrane Gk. chorion = skin & eidos = shape or form* hence membranes around the foetus *adj.- choroid*

chrom- coloured (krohm-)

Chromatin (KROH-mah-tin) the mass of genetic material in the nucleus of a cell, consisting mostly of DNA. It is only visible during interphase.

Chromophore (KRO-moh-for) an organic group on an histology dye which causes the benzene ring on the dye to colour when it attached to Ts.

Chromosome (KRO-moh-sohm) one of the structures (46 in human cells) w/n the cell nucleus that contains genetic material. Chromosomes become visible during cell division.

chron- time (kron-)

Chronic (KRON-ik) long standing (≠ acute), generally used in disease states

chyle- digested fats (KÏ-I) *Gk. = juice.*

cili- eyelash (sil-ee)

Cilium (cil cc um) *Lt cilia – cyelashes* hence hair-like processes associated with cells which is a modification of the CM with specific internal structures as opposed to mv. Ciliary movement generates a flow of fluid (usually mucus) in the extracellular environment. *adj ciliary, ciliated pl cilia*

cine- (sin-ee) movement

Cingulum: *Lt. girdle or belt, adj. cingulate.*

circum- (SER-kum) around , surrounding

Circumcision *Gk cirumcidare = to cut around* **AKA Periotomy** the removal of the foreskin of the penis or clitoris, usually done for religious &/or cultural reasons.
In the female there are a number of variations of this operation:
A - the normal anatomy of the vulva; exposed clitoris prepuce (1), urethral (2), vaginal (3) & anal openings (5)
B - simple removal of the hood of the clitoris (1)- equivalent to male circumcision
C - removal of the clitoris & most of the LMi (4i), obstructing menstral & urine flow (7)
D - infibulation removal of the LMi (4i) sewing together of the LM (4a) leaving only a small opening fluid discharge (8).

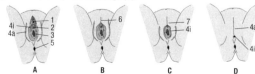

| A | B | C | D |

There are no health benefits to any of these procedures. Diseases of the vulva are increased with the blocking of the menstral & urine discharges & in D childbirth is not possible w/o surgical intervention.

In the male it may protect from certain diseases e.g. AIDS, UTIs & other STDS, & inflammation of the penis. A, B penis before the operation & C after circumcision; showing the removal of the foreskin (1), which in the uncircumcised covers the urethral meatus (2) & in the circumcised exposes the glans penis (3).

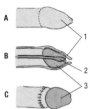

Circumflex: *Lt. circum*= *around*, & *flexere* = *to bend*, hence, bend or bent around.

cirrho- (si-roh) yellow, orange

cis- (sis) on this side

cleist- (klïst-) closed

Cleavage the vertical fold line created when breasts touch, not possible if the breasts are widely spaced or splayed. It is exaggerated when wearing certain bras, &/or breast supports.

clist- closed

Climax AKA Orgasm the peak of any experience which in sexual terms is an orgasm. Exercising the pubococcygeus muscle in both female & male may increase the intensity of the orgasm by increasing the strength of the spasms of the muscular contractions of the climax see Kegal exercises

Climateric AKA Menopause

Clitoridectomy AKA Spay AKA Thelectize removal of the clitoris equivalent of the removal of the penis in the male. This has been done in some cultures for a number of reasons: to reduce the enjoyment of non penetrative SA, including masturbation & lesbianism, *see also Circumscision*.

Clitoris *Gk = key* female equivalent of the male penis - has the same number of N endings & is arguably the most erogenous zone in the female body

Cloquet's fascia membranous layer of the superficial perineal fascia

Cloquet's gland LN in the femoral ring

Cloquet's septum AKA femoral septum

Clue cells cells covered in bacteria which line the wall of the vagina & are a sign of bacterial vaginosis

Clone (KLOHN): *Gk slip* referring to probation by cutting a slip from a plant , hence reproduction & propagation via a single cell

co- (koh) with together

Coagulation (KOH-ag-you-lay-shon) *Lt coaculo = to curdle* as in milk curdling hence the process of clotting turning from a liquid to a solid or semi-solid

Coccyx: *Gk. kokkyx = cuckoo,* whose bill the coccyx resembles, lower bone at the base of the spine, vestigial tail.

Coeliac AS Celiac: *adj. Gk. koilia = belly.*

Coelomic AS Celom

coen- general , common

Coitus AKA Copulation AKA Sexual intercourse AKA Intercourse AKA the Sex Act penetrative SA

> **Coitus analis AKA Buggery, Sodomy** penetrative anal sex - used as a form of contraception, preservation of the hymen & in male to male penetrative intercourse
>
> **Coitus interruptus AKA Coitus reservatus** w/drawal of the penis before ejaculation used by some as a form of contraception &/or safe sex practice
> *adj coital*
> *pre-coital* SA preceding coitus
> *post-coital* SA or feelings associated with coitus after the event

col- with, together

coelom- (SEE-lohm) body cavity

Collagen (KOL-a-jen) a protein that is an abundant component of CT.

Collateral: *adj. Lt. con = together & latus = side,* hence, alongside.

Colliculus: diminutive of *Lt. collis = hill.*

Collum: *Lt. = neck (cf. collar) adj. colli*

Colon (KOH-lun) *Gk. kolon = large intestine* hence the large intestine, a term used interchangeably with the LI

colp- (kohlp) vaginal

Colposuspension surgical technique to "suspend" the vaginal wall and support urinary stress incontinence due to a cystocoele

Columns of Morgagni AKA anal columns

com- together, with

Coma (KOH-mah) Gk koma = sleep hence refers to a depressed state of consciousness & ability to respond to stimuli

Commissure: *Lt. con = together, & missum = sent,* fibres which cross b/n symmetrical parts. generally referring to neural fibres in the brain

con- together with

Conception fertilization and implantation of the blastocyst

Condom a covering of the male or female sex organ to prevent the meeting of the sperm & ova in SA. A barrier contraceptive & barrier against infection: mainly latex coverings for the penis but there are also products for the female & even coverings for oral sex.

Congenital (KON-jen-it-al) present from birth

Connective tissue (kon-EK-tiv Tishh-ew) (CT) one of the 4 basic types of tissue in the body. It is characterized by an abundance of EC material with relatively few cells, and functions in the support & binding of body structures.

contra- opposite against

Continence the ability to contain or control the flow or release of substance c.f. bladder continence (≠ **incontinence**)

Contralateral: *Lt. contra = against, latus = side,* the opposite side (≠ ipsilateral)

Conus (KOH-nus): *Lt. = cone, conus medullaris* - the lower end of the SC.

Convulsions rhythmic spasmodic muscular contraction, which may be normal at climax and is also used for the spasmodic whole body contractions of epilepsy

Cooper's Ligament - occurs in 2 places (1) pectineal ligament; (2) suspensory ligament of the breast

cor- heart

copro- faecal

Corona radiata (kor-ROH-nah ray-dee-AR-tah) several layers of follicle cells that form a protective mantle around the secondary oöcyte.

Coronal (kor-ROH-nal) *Lt. coron = crown,* hence, encircling like a crown the coronal plane extends vertically to divide the body into anterior & posterior portions. AKA the frontal plane *adj coronary, coronoid .*

corp- (kor) body

Corpus: *Lt. = body, pl.- corpora.* pertaining to the body or the main part of the organ

Corpus luteum (KOR-puhs LOO-tee-uhm) a structure w/n the ovary that forms from a ruptured Graafian follicle and functions as an endocrine gland by secreting female Hs.

Corpuscle (KOR-puhs-ehl) *Lt. = a little body* hence used to describe a small body contained w/n a sac, as in red corpuscle (RBC) small package of haemoglobin

Cortex (KOR-tehks) *Lt. = bark, adj. cortical* the outer portion of an organ. (≠ medulla)

cost- (kost) rib *Lt. = rib. adj.- costal*

Cowper's glands AKA bulbourethral glands

Coxa: *Lt. = hip,* hence *os coxae = the hip bone.*

Cramping muscle cramping in the uterus is generally due to the muscles contracting around the arterioles (A) due to prostaglandin release which then causes anoxia and further cramping (B).

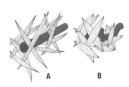

A   B

Cranium (KRAY-nee-um) *Gk. kranion = skull. adj. cranium* consists of all the bones of the skull with the exception of the mandible

Cremaster: *Gk. = suspender*, hence the muscle which suspends the testis.

Crenation (kre-NAY-shun) the shrinkage of a cell caused by contact with an hypotonic solution.

Crescent (KRES-ent) crown of epithelial cells – as seen in glomerulonephritis on Bowman's capsule or around the discharged ovum

-crine (krïn) to secrete

crur- (kroo-r) leg *Lt. = leg, sing crus pl - crura.*

cryo- (krï-oh) cold freezing

crypt- hidden, covered occult

Cryptorchidism congenital absence of one or more testes from the scrotum, un-descended testis / testes

Cunnilingus AKA Oral sex on the female

Curettage the scraping of the uterine cavity often due to a partially missed abortion

cutis - (KEW-tis) skin

Cutaneous (kew-TAY-nee-us) *adj Lt. cutis = skin* the skin.

Cyanosis (SĪ-an –oh-sis): *Gk kyanos –blue material*, hence blueness of the skin, or elsewhere due to the lack of oxygen

Cymbalism AKA Lesbianism

cymbo- (sim-boh) boat shaped

cyrt- bent, curved

cyst-(sist-) sac, bladder

Cyst: (sist-) *Gk. kystis = bladder, adj.- cystic.* cyst referring to fluid enclosed w/in the epidermal layers c.f. an ovarian cyst

Cystoscopy examination of the internal bladder surface via a narrow tube passed through the urethra into the bladder, with a light & camera attached.

cyt-/-cyte (sït-) cell mature cell type

Cytokinesis (SĪ-to-ky-nee-sis) the division of the cytoplasm as a part of the process in mitosis resulting in 2 equal daughter cells.

Cytology (SĪ-tol-oh-jee) the study of individual cells

Cytoplasm (SĬ-to-plazm) the material of a cell located w/n the plasma membrane & outside the nuclear membrane, containing the cellular organelles.

Cytosol (SĬ-toh-sol) the thickened fluid of the cytoplasm. It lies outside the cellular organelle membranes.

Cytoskeleton (sĭ-toh-SKEL-eh-ton) the complex supportive network of microtubules & microfilaments in the cytoplasm

D

dactyl- digit, finger, toe (dak-til)

Dartos: *Gk. = flayed or skinned.* muscle in the skin of the scrotum

de- remove, undoing, reversal, depriving, freeing from

dec- ten , tenth (des)

Decussation (DEE-kus-ay-shon) *Lt. decussatus = crossed like the letter X.*

Deep fascia (FASH-ee-ah) a sheet of CT covering the external surface of a muscle

Deferens: adj. *Lt. = carrying down.*

Degeneration -retrogressive cell & tissue changes short of necrosis

Deglutition: *Lt. deglutire = to swallow,* hence the act of swallowing.

Dehiscence: *Lt. de = away, hiscere = to gape,* hence a separation, a splitting away (as in wounds).

deka- multiple of ten

Deltoid: *adj. Gk. = delta (D),* the capital letter has a triangular shape ▼(c.f. the delta of the Nile)

dem- people, population

demi- (dem-ee) half

Dendrite: or dendron, *Gk. = a tree,* hence like the branches of a tree.

dendro- branching, treelike

Deoxyribonucleic acid (dee-ox-see-rĭ-boh-nyoo-KLAY-ik AH-sid) (DNA) a nucleic acid in the shape of a double helix that contains the genetic information necessary for protein synthesis.

Depress: *Lt. de = prefix implying descent & pressum = pressed,* hence to press down

Depression downward movement or a concavity on a surface.

Dermatome *Gk. derma = skin, tome = a cutting or division,* a segment of skin supplied by a single spinal NR.

derm(o)- skin

dermato- skin

Dermis (DER-mis) *Gk. = skin, adj.- dermal* the layer of the skin lying deep to the epidermis & composed of dense irregular CT. The collagen fibres are maintained by female Hs particularly oestrogen. After the menopause collagen fibres breakdown & the skin appears frailer & translucent as the dermis is reduced.

Detrusor: (DEE-troo-ser) *Lt. detrusio = thrust away.* Muscle of the bladder which contracts & empties it of urine

Detumescence the reduction of a swelling used generally to refer to the return to the normal shape of an erect penis

deuter- secondary, second

di two, twice, double, reversal , separation, apart from

dia- through across, between , apart , complete

Diagnosis (DĬ-ag-noh-sis) (Gk: a deciding – decision) a determination of the nature of the disease

Diaphragm: *Gk. dia = across, & phragma = wall,* hence, a partition, adj. diaphragmatic

Differentiation (DIF-er-ent-she-ay-shon) the process of changing from one kind of tissue or cell to another, generally to a more complex form

Dildo *It. diletto = delight* is a phallus sex toy i.e. one which resembles the penis (generally human) & is used in sexual activity.- This definition does not usually include penile extensions AKA prosthetic penile aids or butt plugs.

diplo- double, twin

Diploid normally each cell has 2 copies of each gene - the diploid state ≠ *Haploid*

dis- apart from, two, twice, double , reversal, separation, difficult, wrong

Discharge AKA Vaginal discharge the term used to imply the oozing of a mucoid liquid generally from the vagina

Discus (DIS-kus): *Lt. = disc. adj. discoid*

Disease (DIZ-eez): *– Eng. dis- ease = lack of comfort,* anything limiting health & comfort of the organism

Distal (DIS-tahl) *Lt. di = apart & stans = standing,* away from the middle of the body or the axis or core of the body (≠ proximal)

Dorsum (DOR-sal) *Lt. dorsum = back adj = dorsal* a directional term indicating toward the back side, or posterior

Douche insertion of a liquid into the vagina or rectum often to clean it or prevent conception but this may disrupt the normal self-cleaning cycle of the vagina, and result in irritation

Douglas fold of - rectouterine fold line of - the arcuate line of the posterior layer of the sheath of the rectus abdominis

Ductus deferens (DUK-tuhs DEF-er-ehnz) AKA Vas Deferens AKA Seminal duct the tube that conducts sperm from the epididymis in the testes to the ejaculatory duct.

duo- (DEW-oh) two

dy- two

dynam- (dĭ-nam) power, energy

dys- (dis) difficult, painful, abnormal

Dyskaryosis the abnormal exfoliated cells of the cervix &/or vagina

Dysmenorrhoea painful periods

Dyspareunia (dis-par-OO-nee-uh) AKA Painful intercourse

Dysphagia: *Gk. dys = difficult & phagein = to eat,* hence, difficulty in swallowing.

Dysplasia changes in the morphology of growing cells / tissues

Dystrophy (DIS-troh-fee) irregular abnormal growth

Dystocia (DIS-toh-see-yuh) *Gk = tokos = childbirth* obstructed labor (≠ Eutocia)

Dysuria pain on urination may occur in association with intercourse in the female & prostatic hypertrophy in the male

E

e- outside external out protrude over away less

ec- outside out to protrude over away less / house

Eccrine (EHK-krin) the common type of sweat gland found all over the body that functions in the maintenance of body temperature.

Eclampsia (EE-klam-see-uh) *Gk eklampsis = shining forth* – convulsions not due to epilepsy or other neural conditions – generally referring to fits in the last trimester of pregnancy due to renal ± hepatic conditions

Ecouteurism an auditory form of voyeurism - listening to the sexual activities of others w/o their consent

Ectasia dilatation or distention of a tubular structure. Maybe physiological & under H influence e.g. duct ectasia of the breast, a dilated milk duct.

ecto- outer out of place

echin- spiny

Ectoderm (EHK-toh-derm) *Gk. ektos = outside & derm = skin* the outermost layer of the 3 primary germ layers in the developing embryo. It gives rise to the NS & to the epidermis & its derivatives

-ectomy to cut out , excise surgically

Ectopic: *Gk. ek = out, and topos = place*, hence out of place.

Edema (eh –DEE-mah) AS Oedema –

Edge: border or margin of a surface.

ef- outside out to protrude over away less

Efferent: *adj. Lt. ex = out, and ferens = carrying*, hence, conducting from

Effluvian (EH-floo-vee-an) shedding of hair, occurs in times of stress & due to H changes e.g, andropause, menopause & pregnancy

Ejaculate the contents of ejaculation

Ejaculation *Lt. ex = out, & jacere = to throw* ejection of semen out of the body, via the urethra generally containing sperm (i.e. male ejaculation) usually accompanied by an orgasm in the male. The initial ejaculate (b/n 10-12 mls) is a thin milky fluid but the final 2-3 mls are thicker possibly to help keep the fluid & sperm inside the female. The consistency & taste of the ejaculate varies with age, diet & frequency of SA. *adj. ejaculatory*

Elasticity (ee-laz-STIS ih-tee) the physiological property of T to return to its original shape after extension or contraction.

Ellis' muscle AKA corrugator cutis ani m.

em- within inside into in on

Emboliformis: *adj. Gk. embolus = wedge or blocking matter.*

Embolus (EM-bohl-us) *Gk embolos = plug*, hence a mass which travels in the BS and suddenly blocks an artery i.e. plugs it up, frequently resulting from a dislodged thrombus. Air emboli are a risk in some forms of SA where air is blown into orifices and there is a defect in the walls of the organs.

Embryo (EHM-bree-oh) *Gk. en = within & bryein = to swell or grow* the early stage of foetal development - in the human this is during the first 8 weeks of life after fertilization.

emet- vomiting

-emia AS –aemia pertaining to blood, generally RBCs

Eminence: *Lt. eminens = projecting*, hence, a projection (usually smooth).

en- within, inside, in, on

Encephalon: *Gk. en = within & kephalos = head*, hence, the brain.

endo- within, inside, into, on

Endocranium: *Gk. en = within, the skull adj. endocranial*

Endocrine: (EHN-do-krihn) *Gk. endo = within: krinein = to separate*, organs that ductlessly secrete products into the BS, generally glands secreting Hs

Endocytosis (ehn'-do-sih-TOH-sihs) the active process of bulk transport of material into a cell. It includes phagocytosis & pinocytosis.

Endoderm (en-DOH-derm) *Gk. endo = within, & derm = skin* one of the 3 primary germ layers in an embryo, it begins as the inner layer, later forms the organs of the alimentary canal (GIT) & the respiratory tract.

Endometrioma a form of endometriosis generally cysts of endometrial T in the ovary

Endometriosis proliferation of the endometrial lining of the uterus in ectopic places

Endometrium (en-doh-MEE-tree-uhm) *Gk. endo = within & metra = uterus pl endometria* the innermost mucosal layer of the uterine wall. The endometrium undergoes changes in response to female Hs, resulting in a 28-day cycle involving menstruation during which 2/3 of the endometrium is sloughed off to be rebuilt again. *pl. endometria*

Endoplasmic reticulum (en-doh-PLAZ-mik reh-TIK-yew-lum) (ER) a cytoplasmic organelle that consists of a series of tubules with a hollow center. It functions in the transport of cellular products (smooth ER), & as a site for protein synthesis (if ribosomes are attached, called rough ER).

Endothelium (en-doh-THEE-lee-um) *Gk. endo = within, & thele = the nipple* a layer of simple squamous epithelium lining the inside of BVs & the heart chambers.

Endotoxin *Gk. endo = within, & toxia = poison adj. endotoxic shock*

Enema fluid inserted or removed from the anus

ent- within inner

enter- to do with the gut , intestines

Enterocoele AS Enterocele a vaginal hernia. Protrusion of the SI into the upper wall of the vagina

Eonism AKA Cross dressing

ep- upon, in addition to, beside among , on the outside , over

epi- upon, in addition to, beside, among, on the outside, over

Epididymis (epi-DID-i-mus) *Gk. epi = upon & didymos = testis* an organ in the male reproductive system that consists of a coiled tube located w/n the scrotum & perched postero-superior to the testis.

episi- (ep-ee-zee) to do with the vulva

Episiotomy (EP-eez-ee-ot-om-mee) the cutting of the vaginal wall to allow the extrusion of the baby when the opening is too small. This should try to avoid the perineal body as the healing of the central lig. is poor & it supports the pelvic structures.

Epispadias urethra opens onto the upper surface of the penis due to incomplete closure (≠ hypospadias on the lower surface)

equi- equal

Erector: *Lt. erectus = straight or upright.*

erg- work

-ergy action

erythr- red

Erotica the depiction of sex in a softer less obvious way than pornography designed to appeal more to females

Erythema (eh-REE-thee-muh) *Gk.: flushing on the skin – redness*

eso- (EE-soh) within

Essayeurs males who have SA with female prostitutes in order to encourage paying customers to become involved as with shills in gambling

Estrue refers to a female animal on heat i.e. the animal is in estrue

eu- good normal well easily

eury- broad wide

Eversion: *Lt. e = out, & versum = turned*, hence turned outwards.

ex- to protrude outside out over away less

Excretion (ek-SKREE-shun) the process by which metabolic waste materials are removed from a cell, a tissue, or an entire body.

Exfoliation (EX-foh-lee-ay-shon) scrapping off or sloughing of the outer epidermal layers – occurring naturally in the vagina & cervix but also in cosmetic procedures to rejuvenate skin on the face & other areas of the body *see also Desquamation*

Exhibitionism sexual excitement from exposing one's body - especially the genitals

exo- outside outer layer out of

Exocrine (EK-soh-krin) gland, one of two main categories of glands, here the cellular products are released into ducts then transported to a body surface or into a body cavity.

Exophilia arousal by the unusual or bizzare

External: *adj. Lt. externus = outward*, hence, further from the inside.

extra- outside of out over beyond, in addition to,

Extracellular environment (EKS-trah-CEL-yew-lar en-VÏ-ROH-ment) the body space outside the plasma membrane of cells.

Extracellular fluid (ECF) the fluid outside the plasma membrane of cells, including interstitial fluid & blood plasma.

Extraperitoneal: *adj. Lt. extra = outside, Gk. peri = around & teinein = stretched*, outside the serous membrane stretched around the inside of the abdominal wall & around the viscera.

F

faci- (fasi) to do with the face

Faecalith (FEE-ku-lith) "faecal stone" – concentration of material in the intestine around fecal material

Fallopian ligament or arch AKA inguinal ligament.

Fallopian tube AKA ovarian tube AKA uterine tube

fasci- (fashi-) band, connection

Fascia (FASH-ee-ah) *Lt. = band or bandage* a sheet or band of dense CT that structurally supports organs and tissues. Deep fascia surrounds muscle, & superficial fascia separates the skin & muscle layers. *adj. fascial*

febri- fever

Fecalith AS Faecalith

Fellatio (fell-AY-shee-oh) AKA irrumation AKA male oral sex *Lt = fellare to suck* oral stimulation of the penis. It is postulated that the original use of lipstick was to advertise the skill & desire of the wearer to perform this practice (*see also Cunnilingus*).

Fetishism sexual satisfaction with an inanimate object or body part

Fetus AS Foetus

Fibroadenoma small solid non-cancerous breast tumours generally occuring in young females

"Fibroid" (FRĪ-broyd) slang term for fibroleiomyoma / fibromyoma – benign proliferation of smooth muscle in the uterus

Fibromyoma the benign proliferation of the smooth muscle of the uterus. There are 3 types: Intramural - in the wall of the uterus 70% (A), Lumenal - growing into the uterine lumen 10% (B) & External 20% (C), fibroids here may be in the cervix (1), broad lig (2), in the serosa (3) or pedunculated (4).

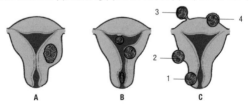

fila- threadlike thread

Fimbria: *Lt. = a fringe, pl fimbriae,* c.f. the finger-like endings of the salpinx which brush the ovary catching the ripe ovum

Fistula (FIST-you-lu) *Lt. = tube* an abnormal opening connecting the inside of an organ to the surface of another

Flagellum (fla-JEHL-um) a single, long extension of a cell composed of protein filaments to provide mobility. In humans, it is found only in sperm cells.

flav- yellow

Flexure: (FLEX-shew-er) *Lt. flexura = a bending.*

Flocculus: *diminutive of Lt. floccus = a tuft.* resembling a picture of a little cloud, with a woolly top & a flat base, c.f. flocculus cerebelli.

Foetus (FEE-tuhs) (FEE-tuhs) the early developmental stage from 8 weeks after fertilization to birth. (AS Foetus) *adj.- foetal.* the early developmental stage from 8 weeks after fertilization to birth. (AS Fetus)

Fold of Douglas AKA rectouterine fold

Folium: *Lt. folium = leaf. pl folia*

Follicle: *Lt. folliculus = a little bag, adj.- follicular.*

Fontanelle: *Fr diminutive of Lt. fons = fountain*, associated with the palpable pulsation of the brain in the anterior fontanelle of an infant.

Foramen (FOR-ay-men) *Lt. = hole. pl. foramina* a natural hole or passage in a bone usually for the transmission of BVs or Ns

Forceps: *Lt. = tongs.*

fore- front or before

Formication sensation of crawling under the skin often associated with menopause

Fornix: *Lt. = arch* hence fornication, because the Roman prostitutes plied their profession beneath the arches of the bridges over the river Tiber.

Foreskin AKA Prepuce the skin around the penis. This may be partially retracted (fr) to show the glans penis & this is removed during male circumcision, while the proximal section is held onto the penis by CT (ff) & fixed anteriorly by the frenulum (f). It is continuous with the skin of the scrotal sac (s) *see also Frenulum*

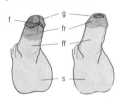

Fossa (FOS-ah) *Lt. = a ditch or trench* hence a depression or concavity on bones or organs formed by several bones

Fovea: *Lt. = a pit* (usually smaller than a fossa).

fract- break

Frenulum: *Lt. = bridle or curb* (diminutive of frenum), it is a CT band which anchors one moving layer to another fixed T e.g. in the mouth & male genitalia it anchors the tongue & penis respectively see also Foreskin.

Frottage AKA Toucherism AKA Haptosis AKA non-consensual rubbing the act of rubbing up against someone with object of sexual arousal often in public, and to the surprise of the unknowing & unwilling subject.

Fundus *Lt. = bottom or base. adj. fundiform* a large, expanded compartment - (note that the fundus of the stomach & uterus are at the top ie they are inverted organs but the fundus of the eye & of the bladder are posterior.

Funiculus: diminutive of *Lt. funis = cord* (used usually for bundles of N fibres).

Furor uterinus AKA Nymphomania

fus- (fewze-) spindle

Fusiform: *adj. Lt. fusus = spindle*, hence, spindle-shaped.

G

G-spot an area which causes sexual arousal when stimulated. It is a roughened circular area on the anterior wall of the vagina in the female, which may cause stimulation of the Skene glands - at the base of the urethra, & female ejaculation (small watery material which is similar to urine).

In the male it is 6-7cm inside & anterior on the rectal wall, roughly at the site of the prostate, and may precipitate an orgasm &/or ejaculation.

Gamete (ga-MEET) a sex cell. It may be male (sperm cell) or female (oocyte). gamma: the 3rd letter of the Gk. alphabet, used in sequence - alpha, beta, gamma, delta, etc.

Ganglion (GANG-lee-ohn) *Gk. = swelling adj.- ganglionic* a cluster of neuron cell bodies located outside the CNS.

Gelatus *Lt = frozen.*

Gendoloma the use of fantasy to accelerate or help with an orgasm

Gemellus: *Lt. diminutive of geminus = twin.*

Gene (JEEN) functional unit of hereditary occupying a specific place on a chromosome, which directs the formation of a specific protein

Genital crisis a bleeding seen in the female baby when the mother's Hs are withdrawn at birth and there is a reactive virginal bleed &/or lactation of the infant breast T

Gerdy's ligament AKA suspensory ligament of the axilla

Germ cells the haploid cell of the species which combines with its opposite to form the zygote in sexual reproduction. Comparison b/n the germ cells of the male & female are listed below.

	Ovum	Sperm
Size	largest cell in the ovary	smallest cell in the testis
Shape	spherical	linear
inner mobility	mobile cytoplasm / Balbiani body	rigid nuclear material
outer mobility	passive	active
Metabolism	active	little activity
Openness	yes	no
Number	1-2 / cycle	millions / ejaculation
produced in	the ovary, inside the body	testes, outside the body
Temperature	warm	relatively cold
when formed	before birth	ongoing from puberty
Age	old	young
formed from - until	before birth - 5 yrs post the commencement of menopause	puberty - death
Maturation	↑ volume	↓ volume
life span	short	long
Easily Stored	No	Yes

Germinal (JER-min-al) epithelium a layer of epithelial cells covering the ovaries.

Gestation (jes-TAY-shun) the period of development prior to birth.

Gestational Diabetes AKA Diabetes of pregnancy

giganto- huge

Gimbemat's ligament AKA lacunar ligament.

Gland *Lt. glans = an acorn, adj.- glandular* a specialization of epithelial tissue to secrete substances. It may consist of a single cell or a multicellular arrangement .

Glands of Littre AKA urethral glands.

Glands of Luschka AKA glomus coccygeum

Gluteal (GLOO-tee-al) *Gk. gloutos = rump or buttock* to do with the rump buttock behind *adj. gluteal, gluteus* **(GLOO-tee-us)**

Glycan (GLĬ-kan) a sugar

Gonad (GOH-nad) *Gk. = reproduction adj. - gonadal* an organ that produces gametes & sex Hs. In the male, it is the testes; in the female, it is the ovaries.

gon- sexual

goni- corner

gnos – *Gk: gnos = to know* **(nos)** *agnos = not to know* **(AG-nos)**

Gravid: *adj.Lt. gravida = pregnant.*

gravis- heavy

Griseum: *adj.Lt. griseus = bluish or pearly grey.*

Gubernaculum: *Lt. something which governs or directs*, like a rudder

Guthrie's muscle AKA sphincter urethrae

gymno- nakedness

gyn- (gĭn-) female

Gynaecomastica development of male breast tissue, present in prepubescent boys but tends to regress with puberty. Re-emerges with age & often particular medications including alcohol, and obesity.

H

Haeme = blood (AS Heme)

Haematocolpos menstral blood in the vagina often due to an imperforate hymen

Haemorrhage (HEM-or-rij) Gk haeme = blood , rhegnymi = to burst forth , hence loss of blood outside the CVS

Haemostasis (heem-oh-STA-sihs) the stoppage of bleeding.

Haemorrhoid: *Gk. haima = blood & rhoia = to flow*, hence likely to bleed. The descent of haemorrhoidal veins out of the anal canal often precipitated by ↑ abdominal P, constipation & anal SA.

Haller's ductulus aberrans AKA diverticulum of the canal of the epididymis

Haller's rete - rete testis

Hand-job tactile stimulation of the male genitalia via hand(s) often until ejaculation.

hapl- single

Haploid term used to describe the genetic component when it has only single copies of each gene/chromosome ≠ *Diploid*

Hegar's sign indication of early pregnancy (6-10weeks) when on vaginal Ex the cervix appears disconnected from the uterus due to early softening

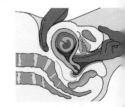

hemi- half

Hermaphrodite AKA Intersex AKA Ambisexual person with the genitalia of both sexes. Generally one set seems to function more than the other & if either are completely developed, there may be normal fertility in that gender.

heter- other different abnormal

Hetaerae highest class of Gk prostitute or female companion

hex- six

Hey's ligament AKA falciform margin of the fascia lata at the saphenous opening

Hiatus (HĪ-ay-tus): *Lt. = a gap* hence a gap in the progress of a process where it is not going up or down

hidr- sweat

Hidrosis (HĪ-droh-sis) disease of the sweat glands

hier- to do with the sacrum

holo- entire

homo- same

homeo (HOHM-ee-oh) same common like

horm- to urge to stimulate

Hormone (HOR-mohn) a substance secreted by endocrine tissue that changes the physiological activity of the target cell.

Hot Flushes *see Vasomotor instability*

hydr- (hĭdr) water

Hydrocephalus: *Gk. hydor = water, koilos = head.* (c.f. cephalic).

Hydrops (HĪ-drops) AKA Oedema

hygr- water

Hymen (HĪ-men): *Gk. = membrane*; generally referring to the membrane across the vagina, pierced by the penis in intercourse. Not all women are born with an intact hymen, so that its presence or absence is not an indication of virginity or its loss.

Hymenorrhaphy AKA Hymenoplasty AKA Hymen reconstruction surgery AKA is the surgical restoration of the hymen.

Hymenotomy the perforation of an imperforate hymen, one which cannot be broken in normal intercourse due to its increased thickness & inelasticity, which causes pain

Hyoid: *adj. Gk. hyoeides = U-shaped.*

hyper - (hĭ-per) excessive ≠ hypo

Hyperchromasia (hĭ-per-KROHM-ay-zee-ya) increased histological staining, of the nuclei often indicative of pathological changes in the tissue / cells

Hyperplasia (HĪ-per-PLAY-zee-ar) an increased production & growth of cells beyond normal limits.

Hypertrophy (hĭ-PER-troh-fee) the abnormal enlargement or growth of a cell, tissue, or organ.

hypo- deficient below under ≠ hyper

Hypoactive uterus AKA Uterus inertia

Hypophysis AKA Pituitary **(HĪ-poh-fif-sis)** *Gk. hypo = down, physis = growth*, hence, a down growth (from the brain). However, this is not the whole truth. Part is an upward growth from the pharynx, *adj.- hypophysial.*

Hypomenorrhea AKA Scanty periods

Hypospadia opening of the urethra on the underside of the penis. This may occur in the glans penis or in the shaft - *see also Epispadia*

Hypothalamus (hĭ-poh-THAL-aw-mus) *Gk. hypo = under, and thalamus* the small, inferior portion of the diencephalon in the brain. It functions mainly in the control of involuntary activities, including endocrine gland regulation, sleep, thirst & hunger.

hyster- (hister-) uterine

Hystero *Gk = hyster* to do with the uterus thought to be the seat of all female emotion hence hysterical

I

iatr- (ee-at-rah) to treat

ictero- (IK-ter-oh) jaundiced

Idiopathic (ID-ee-oh-path- ik) *Gk. = idios one's self, pathos sickness* a spontaneous sickness or illness of unknown origin *(= agnogenic)*

ile - pertaining to the ileum

im- in, into, on, onto, not, non

Imperforate w/o an opening

Implants insertion of material or medication placed w/n a material & inserted into the body or an organ (A) - generally under the skin - dermal (B) or under a muscular (1) layer, sub-muscular (C). Used to enhance or augment the organ as in breast implant (2); or to deliver medication

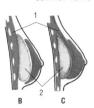

slowly as in depot medication implants which may last up to mnths or years

Impotence the inability to sustain an erection long enough for penetration. Two forms physical & psychological. If the penis is able to become erect throughout the night via involuntary nocturnal erections which occur b/n 3-5 times in the night, then the problem is not physical.

In vitro (ihn VEE-tro) outside the body, such as in a culture bottle.

In vivo (ihn VEE-vo) inside the living body.

infero- low, lower

Incarceration (in-KARS-er-ay-shon) impaction, wedging i.e. incarcerated uterus is trapped behind the Sacrum

Induction to accelerate or brlng on a process c f. induction of labour

Inferior (ihn-FER-ee-or) *Lt. = lower down* a directional term describing a location

Infertility inability to cause conception. In the males this may be due to lack of sperm, or inadequate sperm. in the female this may be due to anovulation or obstruction of the pathway to the ovum; so the sperm does not meet the ovum

Infibulation the scraping out of the fleshy, inner layers of the LM. The remaining outer edges are brought together, hence when the wound heals, the edges fuse together to leave only a pinhole-size opening (A). It forms a thick fibrous scar. This is barely adequate for urination & menstruation, & is inadequate for delivery of a baby. It must be opened when the woman is due to deliver (B).

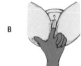

infra- (infruh) below, beneath

Infundibulum (in-fun-DIB-yoo-lum) *Lt. = funnel* the narrow connection b/n the hypothalamus of the brain & the pituitary gland, also, the funnel-shaped distal end of the uterine tube which opens near an ovary.

inguin- (ing-GWIN) pertaining to the groin

Insufflation air introduced into the rectum &/or vagina - SE include severe cramps &/or air embolus.

insul- island

Integument (in-teg-yoo-MENT) *Lt. in = on, tegmen = roof*, hence the skin coat pertaining to the skin & its accessory organs. adj. integumentary

inter- between

Intercellular (in-ter-SEL-yoo-lar) the area b/n cells.

Interstitial cells (in-ter-STIH-shul) cells b/n lobes or structures in an organ e.g. in the testes they are located b/n seminiferous tubules that secrete testosterone, *AKA Leydig cells*.

Interstitial fluid (ihn-tehr-STIH-shool FLOO-id) the portion of ec fluid which fills the T spaces b/n cells. (see also = tissue fluid & intercellular fluid).

Intervertebral disk a cartilaginous joint consisting of a pad of fibrocartilage located b/n two adjacent vertebrae.

Intima: *Lt. = innermost.*

intra- (in-truh) *Lt. = within* **within**

Introitus: *Lt. intro = within, & ire = to go*, i.e. an orifice or point of entry to a cavity or space e.g. vaginal introitus .

Inversion: *Lt. = in, & vertere = to turn*, hence to turn inward, inside out, upside down.

ipsi- same

Ipsilateral: *Lt. ipsi = self, the same, & latus = side*, hence on the same side.

isch- suppression, blocking

Ischaemia (is-KEEM-ee-ya) result of sudden ↓ in the BS to cells or Ts.

ischi- hip

Ischium: *Gk. = ischion = socket*, this bone is so named because the it contributes more than either the Ileum or Pubis to the acetabulum.

Isotonic solution a solution that contains an equal amount of solutes relative to another.

Isthmus: *Gk. = isthmos - a narrow passage.*

K

Kabazzah AKA Kegal exercises the exercising of the pelvic muscles in partic pubococcygeus to strengthen the pelvic floor muscles, vaginal walls & urethral sphincter. Main thrust is to try to hold weights intravaginally or to try to stop urination mid stream, in both males & females. For SA concentrate on the vaginal walls & penile shaft.

Kegal exercises exercises to strengthen the Pubococcygeus m, takes the form of holding something in the vagina - e.g. a pencil or Kegal balls. Strengthening muscles in this area strengthens the whole pelvic floor & may restore continence, particularly in the female after childbirth or menopause.

-kine- move

-kines stimulation of activation for division or growth of cells

Kiss *Eng. cyssan = kiss* pressing of closed lips against another person or object. In SA the kiss used as foreplay & often involves 2 people in with open mouths, tongues & saliva exchange (*cf French kissing*). Kissing has been discussed in this context since the earliest recorded poetry, and ancient Egyptian, and is used in other contexts not discussed here. It has anxiolytic effects & lowers stress & cholesterol.

koilo- hollow concave

Koilocyte is a squamous epithelial cell that has undergone a number of structural changes often secondary to a viral infection or precancerous state, of the anal, cervical (1) &/or vaginal tissue; such as larger, haloed & darkened nuclei (2). These cells are observed in Pap smear preparations along with other changes. Such as : 3 - squamous pearl; 4- regular parakeratosis, 5 - atypical parakeratosis; 6 - atypical keratinized squamous cells; 7 multinucleated macrocyte; 8 -polka dot cell; 9 - balloon cell & 10 - mild metaplasia.

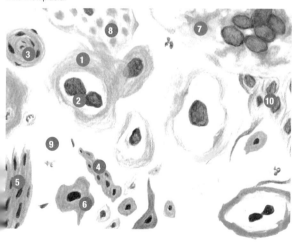

kolp- vagina

Koniocortex: *Gk. konis = dust, and Lt. cortex = bark*, hence, sensory cortex containing mostly granular layers.

Kyphosis (KĬ-foh-sis): *Gk. kyphos = bent or bowed forward*.

L

labi- lip

Labiaplasty surgical modification of the LM ± LMi becoming commoner as a cosmetic technique , but was previously an operation for extended or malformed labia in the vestibule. A before the operation; B with operative markings on the LMi & C the final result with the LMi being smaller than the LM.

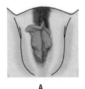 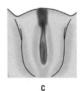

A　　　　　　　　　**B**　　　　　　　　　**C**

Labium (LAY-bee-um) *Lt. = lip pl labia, adj.- labial.* hence a lip and refers to the vulval labia but may refer to the oral labia (lips)

Labrum *Lt. = rim.*

lacri- (LAK-ree) *Lt. lacrima = a tear (drop) lacrimal: adj.* **tear**

Lactation: *Lt. lactans = suckling.* hence, the act of secreting milk.

Lacteal: *adj.Lt. lac = milk, adj lactic* hence, resembling milk.

Lactiferous: *adj. Lt. lac = milk & ferre = to carry.*

Lacuna (lah-KOO-nah) *Lt. lacus = lake* hence, a small pond or gap, adj. *lacunar. pl. - lacunae.*

Lacunae of Morgagni AKA urethral lacunae

lal- talking

lapar- abdominal cavity

lapis- stone

Lata: *Lt. latus = side. adj Lateral* **(LAT-er-awl)** hence nearer the side a directional term describing a structure that is located further from the vertical midline of the body relative to another

Leydig's cells AKA interstitial cells of the testis.

leio- (LǏ-oh) smooth

Leiomyomata AKA Fibroid

Lesion (LEE-zshen) a destructive change in the tissue – such as an inflammation, injury or wound

leuco- white, colourless, pale

Leucorrhoea white discharge from the vagina - if not excessive this is a normal discharge in the self cleaning process of the vagina - too much may indicate an In - the commonest being Candidiasis or yeast infection.

　　　　　　　　　　　　　　　　　　　　© A. L. Neill

leuko- white, colourless, pale

levator- to lift up ≠ depressor

levo- left

Libido (lib-EE-doh) AKA sex drive the urge & interest in having sex

Lieutaud's trigone AKA trigone of the urinary bladder

liga- bind

Ligament (LIG-uh-ment) *Lt. ligamentum = bandage* a band or cord of dense CT that extends from one bone to another -tying it together to provide a joint with structural stability *adj.- ligamentous.*

Line of Douglas AKA the arcuate line of the posterior layer of the sheath of Rectus Abdominis m

linea- (lin-ee-ah) *Lt. = line* line

lingu- tongue *see also* gloss-

 lingua: Lt. = tongue, *adj.lingual.*

Lingual (LIHN-gwal) pertaining to the tongue. For example, the lingual frenulum connects the tongue to the floor of the mouth.

Lingula: diminutive of lingua, hence, a little tongue, *adj.- lingular.*

lio- (LĬ-oh) smooth

lip- fat

lith- stone

Livid *Lt = lividus lead coloured* – discolouration from a contusion or congested pooled blood *adj livedo*

Lochia (LOK-ee-uh) vaginal discharge after giving birth, which continues b/n 4-6 wks postpartum.

Lobe (LOH-b) *Gk. lobos = lobe, adj.- lobar.* roundish projection of any structure

Lobules (lob-YOOL) little lobe

loc- location place

Locus (LOH-kus) *Lt. = a place* (cf. location, locate, dislocate).

longus- long

Lubricants a substance which reduces friction often used with SA. Natural ones include saliva, pre-ejaculate from the male & ungation from the female. Commercial water based lubricants cause the least disruption to the natural environment.

luc- light

Lucidum (LOO-sid-um) *Lt. lucidus = clear.*

lue- syphilis

lumb- loin

Lumbar: *adj.-* lower back *see loin.*

Lumen (LOO-men) *Lt. = opening* the potential space w/n a tubular structure.

Lupus (LOO-pus) - *Gk = wolf* specifically, disease of the skin which is highly destructive and deposits collagenous lesions all over the body –looking like the skin was gnawed

Luteum (LOO-tee-um) *adj. Lt. = yellow.*

ly- dissolved

M

macro- (MAK-roh) big

Macroscopic: *adj.Gk. makros = large, & skopein = to examine*; hence, large enough to be seen with the naked eye, e.g., pertaining to gross anatomy / macroscopic anatomy.

Macrophage (MAK-roh-fahrj) a large phagocytic cell originating from a monocyte.

macula: *Lt. = spot* (cf. immaculate - spotless); *adj.- macular.*

Macule – non-palpable coloured mark on the skin

magna- large, great

Major (MAY-jaw) bigger of the 2 things e.g. Pectoralis major m lying over Pectoralis minor m - bigger & more supf.

mal- abnormal bad

Malignant (MAL-ig-nant) cancerous cells which invade other body parts

Malpighian canal AKA longitudinal duct of the epoophoron

Malpighian layer AKA germinative zone of the epidermis.

Mamma: *Lt. = breast; adj.- mammary.* **(MAM-ar-ree)** a modified sweat gland in the breast that serves as the gland of milk secretion for nourishment of the young

Marcille's triangle contains the Obturator N & is a triangle bounded medially Psoas major m, laterally by the VC & inferiorly by the iliolumbar lig.

Masochism sexual excitement from pain either physical or psychological, inflicted by self or others

mast- pertaining to the breast

Mastectomy removal or 1 or more breasts or parts thereof

Masturbation is self-sexual stimulation, generally of the genitals ± other erogenous zones. This can be done with fingers, hands or objects used to amplify the sexual arousal e.g. sexual toys, *see also Mutual masturbation, Onanism.* Note there is a different pattern in penile masturbation b/n the circumcised & the non circumcised male.

maz- breast

Mazerporosis mutilation of the breasts

meat- opening

Meatus (mee-AY-tus) *Lt. = passage; adj.- meatal* canal, opening passage, particularly if opening onto a body surface as in urinary meatus AKA external urethral orifice - similar to the term orifice

medi- middle intermediate

Medial (MEE-dee-al) *Lt. medius = middle adj medial* a directional term describing a part lying nearer to the vertical midline of the body relative to another part.

Median: *Lt. medianus = in the middle.*

medo- to do with the penis

Medulla (meh-DUL-ah) an inner, or deeper, part of an organ. e.g. the medulla of the kidneys, the medulla of the adrenal gland & the lymph node. ≠ cortex

meg- large

megalo- large

meio- (mǐ-oh) reduced, contraction

Meiosis (MǏ-oh-sis) germ cell division where the genetic material is halved as a device for future fertilization (as opposed to Mitosis)

mel- limb, cheek

melan- black

Melatonin is a H secreted by the pineal gland. It maintains the body's circadian rhythm, ↑ in the dark & ↓ in the light. It is a strong antioxidant, immune system amplifier & helps in the control of female reproductive Hs. Melatonin is a determinant of menarche, the frequency & duration of menstrual cycles, & menopause, *see also Pineal gland.*

Membrane (MEM-brayn) *Lt. membrana = a thin sheet; adj.- membranous* a thin sheet of tissue that lines or covers body structures. It may contain a thin layer of CT ± epithelium

Membranous bone a type of embryonic osseous tissue representing early skeletal development in a late embryo.

men- menses

Menarche the time of the first menstruation

Menopause (men-oh-PORZ) AKA Climacteric - when the ovaries cease to secrete Hs and so menstruation ceases. It is defined as the last menstral period generally 4 yrs after the changes begin to occur in the H cycle & the levels of Oestrogen & Progesterone ↓ due to the failing ovary. Although there may be an abrupt cessation of periods, on average periods continue irregularly for up to 4 yrs before ceasing altogether. Average age of onset 48-52 yo. *see also Premature Ovarian Failure*

Menorrhagia excessive menstral bleeding

Menses AKA Periods

Menstral cup cup to go over the cervix to catch the menstral blood as an alternative to menstral pads or tampons

Menses (MEN-seez) *Lt mensis = month* **AKA Menstruation AKA Catamenia** the material discharged from the vagina during menstruation

ment- mind, chin

mer- part, segment

mes- middle

Mesoderm (MEEZ-oh-derm) *Gk. mesos = middle, & derma = skin* the middle of the three primary germ layers in a developing embryo that forms the muscles, the heart and BVs, & the CT.

Mesothelium (mez-oh-THEE-lee-um) a simple squamous epithelium lining parts of the body's ventral cavity.

Mesosalpinx: *Gk. mesos = middle, & salpinx = tube*; the intermediate part of the broad ligament.

meta- subsequent, transformation, between, changing after

Metrorrhagia irregular uterine bleeding often due to H imbalance (**AKA Breakthrough bleeding**) or at menopause

micro- small

Microvilli (mī-kroh-VIL-ee) microscopic extensions of the cell membrane filled with cytoplasm, ↑ absorptive surface area of the cell.

Micturition (MIK-tyoo-ri-shon): *Lt. micturare = to desire to pass urine.*

mid- middle

Midsagittal (MID-sahg-ih-tal) a plane that extends vertically through the body, dividing it into equal R & L portions *see also parasagittal.*

milli- thousandth

minimus- smallest

Minor- smaller of 2 things e.g. Psoas Minor m lies deep & is smaller than Psoas Major m *see also Major*

mio- reduced contraction

Misandry women who hate men (≠ **Misogyny**)

Misogyny (MIS-oj-en-ee) men who hate women

Mitosis (mī-TOH-sis) the division of a cell's nucleus into two daughter nuclei, each of which contains the same genetic composition as the original parent. When mitosis is followed by cytokinesis, equal division of the whole cell results.

mnem- (mem) memory

Modiolus (MOH-dee-oh-lus) *Lt. a cylindrical borer with a serrated edge*; hence, like a screw; the central stem point of insertion of all the facial muscles around the lips

molar: adj.*Lt. mola = mill.*

Monocyte (MON-oh-sït) a large, agranular WBC that is phagocytic. If the cell moves from the BS to the extracellular tissue, it is called a macrophage.

Mons: *Lt. = mountain*; hence mons pubis, the soft tissue bulge over the pubes, non gender specific term in the female AKA Mons Venutus .

Montgomery's tubercles (glands)
these glands (1) are enlarged
sebaceous glands (2) (found elsewhere
on the breast & skin) & projecting from
the surface of the areola (3)

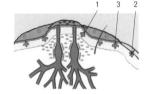

morph- (morf) shape

Morphology: *Gk. morphos = form,*
& logos = word or relation; hence, study of pattern of structure;
adj. morphological.

multi- many

Mutual masturbation generally manual stimulation of the genitals of a partner, with reciprocal stimulation from the other partner with or w/o the use of other objects.

myc- (mïs-) fungal

myel- bone marrow , spinal cord

myo- (mï-oh) muscle

Myocardium (mï-oh-KAHR-dee-um) *Gk. mys = muscle, & kardia = heart,*
adj. myocardial. the primary layer of the heart wall, composed of cardiac muscle tissue.

Myometrium (mï-oh-MEE-tree-um) the smooth muscle layer in the wall of the uterus.

Myotome: *Gk. mys = muscle, & tome = a cutting*; a group of muscles innervated by spinal segment.

myx- (mix) mucoid

Myxoedema AS myxedema (MIX-e-deem-uh) -swelling under the skin due to hypothyroidism – hard oedema (mucoid) in the subcutaneous tissues

N

narc- stupor

necro- (NEK-roh) death

Necrosis (neh-KROH-sihs) death of a cell, a group of cells, or a tissue due to disease.

Negation processes which render a male impotent

neo- (NEE-oh) new

Neonatal: *adj.Gk. neos = new & Lt. natos = born*; hence, new-born.

Neoplasm (NEE-OH-plasm) any abnormal growth of tissue or proliferation of cells not under physiological control – maybe benign or malignant

nephro- renal kidney

neur- nerve

Neuron (NEW-ron) *Gk. neuron = nerve adj.neurium. adj. neural* a cell of NT characterized by its specialization to conduct impulses (conductivity).

neutro- neutral

Niddah AKA Menstral taboo the separation of the sexes around the menstral bleeding time possibly with additional days

noci-(noh-SEE) pain

Nocturnal clitoral tumescence is the female equivalent of the male early morning penile erection, where due to ↑ BF to the area, the clitoris becomes engorged & "erect" This may or may not be associated with feelings of sexual arousal.

Node: *Lt. nodus = knot.*

Nodule diminutive of *Lt. nodus = knot*, hence, a little knot

Norma: *Lt. = pattern or rule, or aspect; adj. normal* according to rule.

nucha- (new-kah-) nape of the neck

Nucha (new-kah-) *Fr nuque = nape or back of the neck; adj.- nuchal.*

Nucleolus (new-klee-OH-lus) a spherical body w/n the nucleus of a cell, not bound by a plasma membrane. It functions in the storage of ribosomal RNA.

Nucleus (NEW-klee-us) *Lt. = kernel or nut* the largest structure in a cell. It contains the genetic material to determine protein structure & function, the DNA. It is enveloped by a double-layered plasma membrane.

null- none

Nulliparous *adj* describes a woman who has not had a birth

Nymphotomy the removal of the LMi to reduce the size of the vaginal orifice for SA.

O

O'Beirne's sphincter circular muscle fibers at the junction of the sigmoid colon & rectum

ob- against , in front of

Obturator: *Lt. obturatus = stopped up*; hence a structure which closes a hole.

oc- against in front of

Occult hidden

oedem- (er-DEEM-) swelling (AS edem-)

Oedema pathological swelling of an organ or region

Oestrus AS Estrus (EE-strus) the time in the menstral cycle of greatest fertility - in humans this is 2-3 days prior to ovulation

-oid like

olig- scant deficient few little

Oligomennorrhoea minimal menstral bleeding < 20mls

-ology (o-loh-jee) study of

-oma tumor or lump

Onanism archaic term for masturbation and may be used for Corpus Interruptus - i.e. withdrawing the penis prior to ejaculation as a form of contraception

Oncogene (ON-ko-jeen) a gene that can transform the cell into an oöcyte

Ontogeny (ON-toj-en-ee) development of an individual growth pattern

Oöcyte (OH-oh-sït) AKA Ovum, egg a gamete produced w/n an ovary.

or- ora- *Lt. ora = margin or edge* **mouth**

Oöphorectomy surgical removal of the ovaries

Oral caressing refers to anything to do with kissing, licking, nibbling, sucking & other nonspecific but generally stimulating actions, which involve the lips, mouth, teeth &/or tongue

Organ a group of tissues & cells which arc bound together to perform a specific function

Organ of Giraldes AKA paradidymis.

Organelle (or-gan-EL) a component of a cell that has a consistent, similar structure in other cells & performs a particular function

Orgasm intense paroxysmal emotional excitement, the climax of SA towards the end of coitus usually accompanied by ejaculation in the male
Four types discussed
    Plateau - involving the whole body in excitement w/o ejaculation or tumescence
    Tonic - involving the genital area & pelvic muscles

Clonic - involving the genital area & pelvic muscles & ejaculation

Fusional - an involvement of more than one site in the excitement

Orgy AKA Group Sex

Orifice (or-EE-fiss) an opening especially into the mouth or a cavity e.g. urethral orifice AKA external urethral orifice *see also Meatus*

ortho- (or-thoh) straight straightening

-osis condition of / disease of – non-inflammatory

Oscultation AKA Kiss (oral)

Ossify: *Lt. os = bone, & facio = make*; to form bone & ossification, the process of forming bone

osteo (os-TEE-oh) pertaining to bone

Osteopenia moderate loss of bone which is reversible. Bone trabeculae are not lost, only thinned at this stage and can be restored, with diet & exercise

Osteoporosis significant loss of bone, including loss of bone trabeculae, which is not reversible & leads to pathological fractures. This is a symptom of menopause, particularly in the axial skeleton.

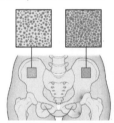

-osteum (os-tee-um) pertaining to bone

Ovary (OH-vahr-ee) *Lt. ovum = egg pl - ova* the female gonad, or primary reproductive organ that produces gametes & female sex

Oviduct AKA Ovarian duct AKA Fallopian tube AKA Uterine tube AKA Salpinx

Ovulation the release of the oöcyte from the ovary from a mature follicle

Ovum AKA Öocyte AKA Egg *pl ova*

oxy- (OKS-ee) sharp

P

paed- child

pali- recurrence

pan- general overall

Pansexuality AKA Omnisexuality *Gk pan = all & omin= every*: is sexual attraction toward people of all gender identities & biological sexes. It may be considered as a separate sexual orientation, where there is no recognition of any form of gender difference / gender blind *see also Bisexuality.*

Papilla (paw-PIHL-ah) *Lt. = nipple or teat; adj.- papillary* a small finger-shaped projection.

par- beside

para- against aside abnormal unequal

Paradidymis: *Gk. para = beside of near & didymis = twinned or paired*, refers to testes; the collection of convoluted tubules in the spermatic cord, above the head of the epididymis.

Paraesthesia: (PA-rah-theez-ee-uh) *Gk. para = beside, & aisthesia = sensation*; abnormal sensation, e.g. burning or pricking.

Paralysis: (PA-ral-i-sis) *Gk. para = beside, near, lyein = to loosen*; loss or impairment of muscle function.

Parametrium (Pa-rah-MEET-tree-um) *Gk. para = beside, & metra = womb*; CT w/n the broad ligament alongside the uterus.

Parasagittal unequal vertical divisions b/n R & L in the body *see also Sagittal & Midsagittal*

Parenchyma (pa-REN-kïm-ah) *Gk para = beside or near, en = in & chein = to pour* the functioning elements of an organ as opposed to the structural or supporting elements (≠ stroma)

Paresis (Pa-REE-SIS): *Gk. = relaxation*, but has come to mean partial paralysis.

Parietal (pa-RÏ-eh-tal) *Lt. parietalis, pertaining to paries = wall* pertaining to the outer wall of a cavity or organ i.e. parietal layer of the pericardium outer of the 2 layers of the pericardium (≠ visceral).

Parous: Lt. pario = I bear (children); applied to women who have borne children ≠ nulliparous,

Pars: *Lt. = part.*

part- childbirth

Paruresis (PAR-yoo-ree-sis) fear of urinating in public, more difficult for a male particularly in the urinals of public toilets, & for females in cubicles w/o doors. It is not directly related to sexual dysfunction either physiological or psychological.

path-/ -pathy disease / disease of

Pathogenesis – origin or cause of a disease

Pathology (path-ol-LOH-jee) the study or science of diseases.

Pawlik's triangle an area on the ant. wall of the vagina in contact with the base of the bladder, which is w/o the normal vaginal rugae

Pectus carinatum AKA Barrel chest AKA Pigeon chest

Pectus excavatum AKA Hollow chest

Pelvis: *Lt. = basin, adj.- pelvic.*

Penetrative sex AKA Inner sex (≠ Outer sex, Non-penetrative sex) forms of the sex act which involve 2 or more persons - e.g. anal sex, fingering, oral sex in which one inserts something organic or otherwise into an orifice of a partner

Penis (PEE-nihs) *Lt. = tail*, the male organ of copulation through which most of the urethra extends. (cf. appendix, appendage).

-penia (PEEN-ee-uh) lack of

per- through, excessive

peri- around, about, beyond

Perianal *Gk. peri = around, & Lt. anus = lower opening of alimentary canal.*

Perimenopause the period b/n the cessation of the periods for a year (the menopause) & the onset of hormonal symptoms, which may be up to 3 yrs long & may extend into the menopause

Perineal body AKA Central lig.

Perineum: *Gk. peri = around & neum = birth* - hence around the natal area, the caudal aspect of the trunk b/n the thighs or the region of the trunk below the pelvis *adj perineal*

Peristalsis: *Gk. peri = around & stellein - to constrict*; a circular constriction passing as a wave along a muscular tube; *adj.- peristaltic.*

Peritoneum (per-it-on-NEE-um) *Gk. periteino = to stretch around* the extensive serous membrane associated with the abdominopelvic cavity. *adj.- peritoneal.*

pero- stunted, malformed

Pessary a device to restore the position of the pelvic contents when they have prolapsed

Petit's ligaments AKA uterosacral ligaments

Phallus (FA-lus): *Gk. phallos = penis.*

physi- (FIZ-ee) natural

Placenta (pla-SEN-tar) *Lt. = a flat, round cake.* The filter separating the mother from the growing baby in the uterus

plan- flat level, to wander

-plasia (FAY-zee-uh) growth

plat- broad flat

pleo- (PLEE-oh) many

pleur- (PLER) lungs respiratory

Pleura (PLEW-rah) *Gk. = a rib* but has not come to mean the serous membrane lining the lungs (visceral layer) & inner rib & intercostal surfaces (parietal layer) associated with the lungs

Plexus (PLEKS-uhs) *Lt. = a network or plait.* a network of interconnecting Ns, veins, or lymphatic vessels

pluri- several

poikilo- (POYK-il-oh) irregular

polio- (POH-lee-oh) grey

poly- (POL-ee) many

Polyp (PO-lip) structure with stalk & rounded, swollen head, generally benign

por- passageway

postero- posterior part

Posterior (pos-TEE-ree-or) *Lt. post = behind (in place or time).* a directional term describing the location of a part being toward the back or rear side relative to another part.

Posterior pituitary gland AKA Neurohypophysis the part of the pituitary gland at the base of the brain consisting of the axons of neurons originating in the hypothalamus & supporting tissue

Pouch of Douglas AKA rectouterine pouch

Poupart's ligament AKA inguinal ligament.

prae- in front of, before

pre- in front of before

Premature ovarian failure shutdown or failure of the ovarian function < 40yo occurs in 1% of females. Aetiologies - autoimmune, genetic

Premenstrual syndrome syndrome of tenseness & irritability prior to the menstral bleeding

Prepuce: *Lt. praeputium = foreskin* of penis or clitoris.

presby- old

Priapism permanently erect penis in young boys

prim- first

Primagravida first time pregnancy

Primary germ layer one of 3 layers of cells that differentiate during the embryonic stage to give rise to all tissues in the body. They are the endoderm, mesoderm & ectoderm.

pro- in front of

Process (PROH-sehs): *Lt. = going forwards, indicating growing out, i.e. an outgrowth,* general term used to describe any marked projection or prominence usually bone

proct- anus rectum

Proctitis (PROK-tĭ-tis) inflammation of the anus &/or lower part of the intestine i.e. rectum (last 10cm of the large bowel) SS pain on bowel movements; soreness in the anal & rectal regions; feeling of incompletion after a bowel movement, tenesmus; haemorrhoids; bleeding &/or discharge from the anus. The commonest cause is trauma to the anal area or infection generally via anal intercourse (generally an STD)

Prognosis (prog-NOH-sis) *Gk pro- = in front of & gno- = to know – fore knowledge* hence the expected outcome of a disease

Prolapse (PROH-laps) to slip & fall out of place

Prone (pr-ohn) face down, recumbent face-down posture.

Pronate: *Lt. pronatus = bent forwards*; to pronate = to turn the hand so that the palm faces downwards or posteriorly ≠ supine.

Prostate (PROS-stayt) gland *Gk. pro = before, & Lt. = statum = stood* something which stands before – e.g. the prostate gland stands before the urinary bladder. A walnut-shaped gland surrounding the urethra as it emerges from the urinary bladder in males. Its secretions contribute to semen.

Proximal (PROKS-i-mal) *Lt. proxime = nearest* a directional term indicating a body part that is located nearer to the origin or point of attachment to the trunk than another; opposite of distal

Pruritis itching

Pruritis vulvae itching and irritability of the vulval area.

pseudo- (syoo-doh) false

Pseudocyesis AKA False pregnancy AKA Phantom pregnancy

Psoas: *Gk. = loin.*

Puberty: *Lt. puber = adult*; hence, the time when hair appears in the pubic region - i.e., near the pubis - as a secondary sexual characteristic.

Pubes (pewbs): *Lt. = adult or signs of manhood*, hence the lower abdominal secondary sexual hair.

Pubic symphysis diastasis movement of the PS in pregnancy

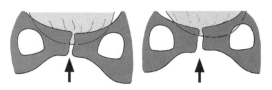

Pudendal: *Lt. pudendus = shameful*; hence, pertaining to the external genitalia.

Puerperium (pyoo-POO-ree-um): *Lt. puerpera = woman in the childbed* the time of childbirth to the time when the uterus returns to its normal size; ~6 weeks postpartum, postpartum period adj peurperal

pyelo- basin , pelvis (generally renal pelvis)

pykno- thick, dense

pyo- pus

Q

Quickening feeling of the foetal movements in pregnancy generally at about 18wks

R

rami- (ray-mee) branch

Ramus: *Lt. = branch*; hence, a branch of a nerve, bone or blood vessel.

Raphe: *Gk. = a seam*; hence, the line of junction of the edges of 2 muscles or areas of skin.

re- return, back again

Rectum: *Lt. rectus = straight.* The rectum was named in animals where it is straight - not so in Man

Region (REE-jon) an area often of the abdomen defined by anatomical surface markers, used to enter the abdomen or to locate pain or an abnormality smaller than a zone or zona.

ren- kidney

Rete (REE-tee): *Lt. = a net; adj. reticular.* hence, a network of veins or tubules.

retro- *prefix Lt. = backwards.* **located behind**

Retroflexion: *Lt. retro = backwards, & flexion = bent*; the position of being bent backwards, applied to the angulation of the body of the uterus on the cervix.

Retroversion: *Lt. retro = backwards, & version = turned*; the position of being turned backwards, applied to the angulation of the cervix uteri on the vagina.

rhe- flow

rheum- mucoid or watery discharge / relating to joint pain

rhod- red

rigor- *Lt rigor = stiffness*

Ruga (ROO-gu) *Lt. ruga = a wrinkle*, hence, wrinkled. *pl. – rugae; adj. – rugose* used to describe the horizontal folds of the mm in the vagina

S

Sadism sexual excitement from inflicting pain on another either physical or psychological

Safe sex SA which use devices to stop any In from being passed from one person to another & does not involve harmful practices that could result in bodily harm to the members involved in the activity

salping- tube

Salpinx (SAL-pinks): *Gk. = trumpet*; the uterine (ovarian) or auditory tubes, each of which is trumpet-shaped. *pl Salpinges* **(sal-pin-JEES)**

Saphenous *Gk. saphenes = obviously visible.* The saphenous veins become obvious when varicose.

scel- leg

schiz- split

Scopophilia a form of voyeurism but often with the consent of those who are being watched

Scrotum: possibly derived from *Lt. scorteus = leather; adj.- scrotal.* the skin sac which encloses the testicles & VD. Any fluids present as a result of injury etc. are normally resorbed over 3 days

Sexual abuse unlawful carnal knowledge of a woman / man by force, fear or fraud.

Secrete: (seh-KREET) *Lt. secretus = separated*; hence, to produce a chemical substance by glandular activity *adj. secretory; noun, secretion.*

Semen: *Lt. = seed; adj. seminal* (seminal vesicle).

semi- half partial

seps- decay

Septum: *Lt. saeptum = fenced in*; hence, a dividing fence or partition- generally of CT.

Serosa (ser-OH-suh) AKA Serous membrane *Lt. = like serum, serum- like* any serous membrane. (also, the outer membranous layer of a visceral organ containing BS & NS as well as lymphatic drainage), similar to the capsule of an organ.

Sexercise slang term for sex being used as exercise - so it tends to use the more vigorous sex positions of sexual intercourse & interplay. Many forms of sex play are good exercise for the MSS & cardiovascular system. It has also been postulated that it acts to stimulate mental abilities. Note many sex positions allow for adaptation for most body systems to be exercised quite vigorously.

The average sexual intercourse session burn as many calories as that of a short walk ~69 cals

Sexual Drive is the sum of a person's desire to have sex combined with their ability to do so

Sexual position the position in which sexual play including penile & vaginal intercourse occurs.

Sex toys devices used in SA

Sexuality is the sum of a person's attitudes, behaviours, experience, inherited characteristics & knowledge wrt how they relate to being either male or female. This includes their psychological perceptions as well as their physicality.

Shrimping the tasting/sucking of toes in a sexual way ± sauces

Sigmoid: *adj.Gk. sigma= S-shaped*, hence, S-shaped.

Skene's gland it is from this gland that the female can "cum" & ejaculate in some cases

Smegma creamy odiferous substance produced at the base of the glans penis & the glans of the clitoris (much less in the female & circumcised male).

Soma (SOH-mah) *Gk. = the body adj.* somatic pertaining to the body or the main part of an organ or a cell but not the viscera

Somite: *Gk. soma = body*, hence an embryonic body segment

Sonohysterography installation of the saline into the uterine cavity (generally to detect masses in the cavity used with US)

Spasm: *Gk. spasmos = an involuntary contraction of a muscle; adj. - spastic, or spasmodic.*

Sperma: *Gk. = seed or semen, adj. spermatic.*

Spermatozoa AKA Sperm cells. They are the formed male gametes produced by meiosis from cells w/n the walls of seminiferous tubules of the testes. Individual spermatozoa are capable of locomotion due to the presence of a single flagellum.

Spermatic cord (spehr-MAH-tik kord) a narrow bundle of tissue in the male reproductive system extending from the epididymis to the inguinal canal, consisting of the ductus deferens, cremaster muscle, BVs, lymphatics, nerves, & CT.

sphen- wedge

Sphincter (SVINK-ter) *Gk. sphinkter = a tight binder*; i.e. a circular muscle which closes an orifice; *adj.- sphincteric.*

spir- coiled, respiration, breath

Spooning intimate position where the couple form a spoon - by bending into each other - generally with the ale or taller person on the outside

stas- stopped

steat- (STEE-at) fat

steno- narrow

Stereocilia: *Gk. stereos = solid, & cilium = eyelash*, hence non-motile microvilli.

Sternum: *Gk. sternon = chest or breast; adj. sternal.*

Stenosis (STEN-oh-sis) *Gk = narrowing* hence narrowing of a duct, BV or other passage

Stoma: *Gk. = a mouth.*

Stratum *Lt. = a covering sheet, or layer.* generally referring to the skin layers pertaining to a multiple-layered arrangement *adj. - stratified*

Striae AKA Stretch marks common acquired condition of the skin, presents as parallel bands of discoloration on the skin, associated with growth spurts or rapid weight gain, as in pregnancy. Initially bright red or deep purple they gradually fade to atrophic white bands which are permanent. When forming they may itch but are often asymptomatic, & they thin & weaken the epidermis (E), reduce the depth and number of dermal papillae (P) & places the collagen closer to the surface (Sc), forming a separation b/n the skin with dermal papillae & the thinner stretched striae (S).

Striae Gravidarum – stretch marks of pregnancy often with a single midline striae Linea Nigra (LN)

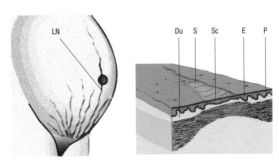

Stroma (STROH-mah) *Gk. = bed or mattress* supporting bed of cells, CT or matrix upon which the parenchyma builds

sub- under less than partial

sud- sweat

Sudoriferous (syoo'-dor-IF-er-us) gland an exocrine gland located in the skin that secretes sweat. (also = sweat gland).

Sudomotor: *Lt. sudor = sweat, and movere = to move*, hence stimulate the sweat glands.

suf- under

super- over

Superficial (soo-per-FISH-al) *Lt. super = above & facies = surface*; hence, nearer the surface. a directional term indicating the location of a part that is toward or nearer to the body surface relative to another (≠ deep).

Superior (soo-PEER-ee-or) AKA craniad AKA Cephalad *Lt. superus = above* a directional term indicating the location of a part that is nearer to the head region than another.

Supination: *Lt. supinus = recumbent on the back* the act of turning the back of the hand to face posteriorly; verb - supinate ≠ pronate. adj. - supine

supra- *Lt. prefix = superior to* **above over**

Suture (SEWT-jah) *Lt. sutura = a seam* the saw-like edge of a cranial bone that serves as a joint b/n bones of the skull; the stitching of 2 opposing edges of tissue.

sym- together union association

Symmastia AS Symnastia (SIM-mast-ee-ya) when the breast T from one side is connected to that of the other side - generally congenital

Symphysis (SIM-fi-sis): *Gk. syn = with & physis = growth*; a joint - bone + fibrocartilage + bone generally used for joints in the median plane, often fuse later in life e.g. the pubic symphysis.

syn- the close proximity of, or fusion of 2 structures

Synapse (sïn-APS) *Gk. syn = with, & aptein = to join* the junction b/n the axon of one neuron & the dendrite or cell body of another neuron. It is the zone of the passage of the impulse from one neuron to another

Syncytium: *Gk. syn = with & kytos = cell*, a multinucleate mass of protoplasm formed by cells merging as in Giant cells & the outer syncytium of the placenta

Syndrome: *Gk. syn = with, & dromos = running*; i.e. a group of signs and symptoms, characteristic of a certain pathology.

T

Tantra *Sanskrit web of life* an Eastern philosophy concerned with experiencing fully the pleasures of the moment - this includes sexual pleasure & has as its aim the enjoyment of the sexual journey with or w/o the end result of an orgasm

tect- covering

Tectum *Lt. tectorium = roof adj tectorial* hence an overlying surface

Tenesmus (TEN-ez-mus) AKA Rectal tenesmus *Lt teinem = to stretch* the feeling of a full bowel & the continuing need to defecate even when the bowel is empty (may also be applied to the bladder i.e. *vesicular tenesmus*). This is often associated with other bowel diseases including proctitis.

terato- abnormal or monstrous growth

Teres: *Lt. = rounded, cylindrical.*

Testicle: *Lt. testiculus = the male gonad* (see testis).

Testis (TEHS-tihs): *Lt. testiculus = the male gonad. Lt. testis = a witness. pl. - testes* one of a pair of male gonads (sex glands) located w/n the scrotum that produces sperm cells & testosterone. Under Roman law, no man could bear witness (*testify*) unless he possessed both testes.

Testosterone a steroidal H secreted by interstitial cells (cells of Leydig) located w/n the testes. It promotes the development of male secondary sex characteristics & the development of spermatozoa. It peaks at 18yo in most males ↓ @ 1% per year. If there is a sudden larger ↓ there may be symptoms *see also Andropause*

terti (ter-shi-) third

Tetralogy: *Gk. tetra = four, & logos = discourse, combination of 4 elements* e.g. symptoms or defects.

Theca: *Gk. theka = a capsule, sheath.*

Thrombus a blood clot that has formed & is attached to a vein or artery.

Thyroid: *Gk. thyreos = shield, & eidos = shape or form*; shaped like a shield (shields the glottis).

Tissue (TI-shoo) a group of similar cells that combine to form a common function.

Titooing semi-permanent tattoos on the nipples to change their shapes

Tongue (tung) the muscular organ of the digestive system that is anchored to the floor of the mouth and wall of the pharynx. It plays major roles in swallowing & speech formation.

Totipotent refers to a cell which is truly able to transform itself into any other cell - used to be thought that this was only the germ cells of the body - but it is now possible to transform many of the other cells in the body to this form - *stem cells*

Touch discrimination 2 point touch discrimination is a measure of the number of N endings present in a particular region, the closer, the denser & more sensitive the area comparing different sites it can be seen that the tongue tip actually has the greatest number of nerve endings/mm^2

Body part	# mms
Anus	4-5
Clitoris	3-4
Glans penis	
Pre-tumescent	5-9
Tumescence	9-15
Post-tumescent	3-4
Lips	4-5
Neck	50-60
Nipple (Breast)	8-10
Tongue - tip	1-2

trans- crossing changing

Transgender a person who identifies with the opposite sex but has not undergone a transforming operation - keeping the original genitals

Transsexual a person who identifies with the opposite sex & has undergone a transforming operation

Transvestite a person who is aroused by cross dressing

Transitional epithelium a type of epithelial tissue characterized by its ability to expand in size and recoil, giving the organs it lines a feature of elasticity. Transitional epithelium forms the inner lining of the urinary bladder & ureters

Transudate extravascular fluid of low specific gravity often resulting from ↑ P or engorgement of the vessels & appearing as small sweat-like droplets e.g. vaginal transudation where small droplets appear in the vagina when the BVs are engorged due to arousal

Transvestism Sexual excitement & gratification from wearing the clothes of & acting in the manner of the opposite sex

Trauma (TRAW-mah) *Gk injury*, wound physical or psychological

tri- three

Trocar (TROH-kar) instrument used to access internal cavities e.g. the full bladder

trocho- round

trop- turn change

troph- (TROHF) nutrition

Tumor AS Tumour: (TEW-mah) *Lt. tumere = to swell* indicating an inflammatory process (fluid swelling) or a neoplasm when the swelling is from new cellular growth

Tunica (TEW-nik-uh): *Lt. = shirt*; hence a covering, generally referring to layers around an organ or T.

© A. L. Neill

U

Ulcer (UL-ser) *Lt ulcus = wound, sore*, hence lack of continuity on the skin - must penetrate all the layers of the skin

Ungation fluid from the vagina to lubricate it during SA

uni- first one

Urachus: *Gk. ouron = urine, & echein = to hold*, the canal connecting the foetal bladder & umbilicus.

Ureter (YEW-ree-tar) *Gk. oureter = passage from kidney to bladder* a long, narrow muscular tube extending from the kidney to the urinary bladder & transports urine using gravity & peristalsis.

Urethra (yew-REE-thrah) *Gk. ourethra = passage from bladder to exterior* a tube extending from the urinary bladder to the exterior; carries urine in females and urine & semen in males.

Uterus: (YEW-tehr-uhs) *Lt. = womb.* a hollow muscular organ in the female reproductive system that serves as a site of embryo implantation, development & menstruation.

Utricle: diminutive of *Lt. uterus = womb.*

Urinary bladder (yew-rin-AR-ee BLAD-ar) AKA Bladder a hollow muscular organ located at the floor of the pelvic cavity that temporarily stores urine.

Uterine tube (YEW-tehr-ihn toob) AKA Fallopian tubes AKA oviducts one of 2 tubes that transport ova from the ovaries to the uterus in the female reproductive system.

V

Vagina (vaj-Ĭ-nuh) *Lt. = sheath; hence, invagination is the acquisition of a sheath by pushing inwards into a membrane*, a tubular, muscular organ of the female reproductive system extending b/n the vulva & the uterus & evagination is similar but produced by pushing outwards. **adj. vaginal**

Vaginal Discharge is any fluid / material oozing from the vagina - normal may be clear, white , yellow ± white flecks & may ↓ mid-cycle & become ↑ viscous. The pH is generally acidic (~4.3) which prevents Ins in the vagina. Any changes may indicate In in this area

Vaginismus (VAJ-in-is-mus) involuntary spasms of the vaginal wall associated with penile penetration

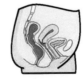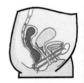

Vaginosis diseases of the vagina

Vanilla sex sex which does not involve elements of BDSM and includes the practices of most western heterosexual couples

Varicocoele (VA-rik-OH-seel): *Lt. varix = vein & Gk. kele = tumour*, a varicose condition of the veins of the pampiniform plexus.

Varix (VAR-ix): *Lt = dilated vein*

Vas deferens AKA Ductus deferens. It is a tube extending b/n the epididymis & the urethra in the male that conveys spermatozoa during ejaculation.

vaso- pertaining to BF

Vasomotor instability BVs in particular skin arterioles become unstable and allow for a sudden ↑ in the dermal BF, causing flushing & heat - generally the cause of *hot flushes* experienced in menopause

Vascular (VAS-kyew-lar) *Lt. vasculum, diminutive of vas*; hence, pertaining or containing BVs.

Vein (vayn) a BV that transports blood from body tissues to the heart. *adj. - venous*

ven- vein

Venipuncture (VEEN-EE–punc-tewr) puncturing of a vein – (in order to take a blood sample)

Venter: *Lt. = belly*; hence, ventral, pertaining to the belly side. adj. - ventral

Ventral a directional term describing the location of a part nearer to the anterior or front side of the body relative to another.

Vermiform: *Lt. vermis = a worm, and forma = shape*; hence, worm-shaped.

Verruca (ve-ROO-kuh): wart

vesic- to do with the bladder

Vesica: *Lt. = bladder, adj.- vesical*

Vesicle (VEEZ-i-kel) *diminutive of Lt. vesica = bladder, hence a little bladder* a small sac containing a fluid. In the cell, it is a membranous sac w/n the cytoplasm which contains cellular products or waste materials, and creates a microenvironment w/n the cell (*see also organelle*).

Vesicula: diminutive of *Lt. vesica = bladder; seminal vesicle.*

Vestibule (VEHS-tih-byewl) *Lt. vestibulum = entrance hall* a small space that opens into a larger cavity or canal. A vestibule is found in the inner ear, mouth, nose & vagina.

Visceral (VIHS-er-ahl) *Lt. viscus = an internal organ* pertaining to the internal components (mainly the organs) of a body cavity; pertaining to the outer surface of an internal organ ≠ parietal.

Visceral peritoneum (VIHS-er-ahl per-ih-toh-NEE-uhm) a serous membrane covering the surfaces of abdominal organs.

Viscus: *Lt. = an internal organ, pl. - viscera, adj.- visceral.*

Vital: *Lt. vita = life.*

Vitelline: *Lt. vitellus = yolk.*

Vitreous: *Lt. vitreus = glassy.*

vivi- alive

volv- turn

Voyeurism sexual excitement from viewing other's sexuality

Vulgar: *Lt vulgaris = usual*; common, plentiful

Vulva: *Lt. = the external female genitalia.*

Vulvar vestibularitis inflammation of the vulval area

W

Womb AKA Uterus

X

xanth- yellow

xen- different

xero- (ZAIR-roh) dry

Z

Zona (ZOH-nah) *Lt. = a belt; hence, a circular band* an area smaller than a region in an organ as in the adrenal gland

Zonule: diminutive of zona.

Zoophilia sexual excitement from intercourse with animals

Zoster: *Lt girdle*

zyg- yoke

-zyme enzyme

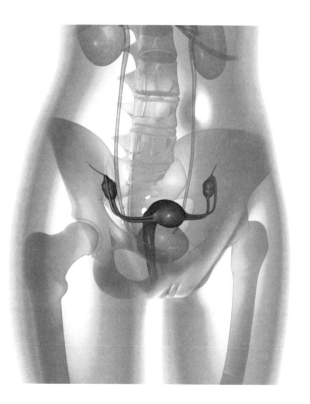

Abortion AKA Miscarriage

A Threatened Abortion - painless vaginal bleeding

B Inevitable Abortion - bleeding + contractions

C Incomplete Abortion - bleeding + contractions + contents

D Contents of a Complete Abortion

E US of the Uterine Cavity after a Complete Abortion

F Missed Abortion - foetal death w/o expulsion

G Changes of a Missed Abortion - failure of uterine growth

An Abortion is the termination of a pregnancy by the removal or expulsion from the uterus of its contents before viability. If this occurs spontaneously it is generally referred to as a miscarriage.

Spontaneous abortions in the early weeks (0-10) are generally due to ovofoetal problems whereas later ones are due to maternal factors.

If an abortion is missed the woman may not be aware that the foetus has died, but her uterus will not continue to grow.

1   18 wk profile

2   14 wk profile - flat abdomen

3   18 wk foetus - died at 14 wks so has remained the same size

4   no loss of uterine contents

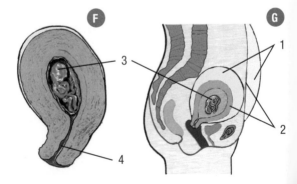

© A. L. Nei

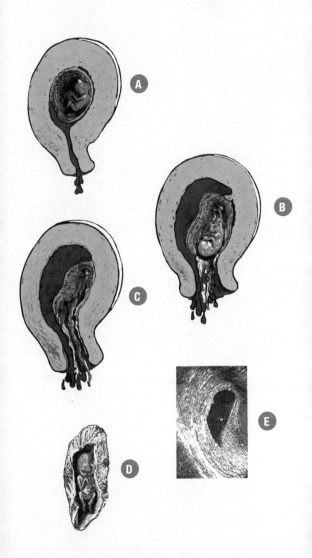

Birth
Lie & Presentation

Macroscopic view
A longitudinal lie
    b   Breech 4%
    c   Cephalic 95%
B oblique lie 0.5%
C transverse lie 0.5%

The lie of the foetus refers to the axis of the foetus compared to that of the mother - and the presentation the part which is in the lower part of the uterus. The attitude of the foetus is generally flexed - i.e. all the limbs are flexed - but occasionally it may be that limbs are extended particularly in breech presentations. Note that these positions are not important until labour is established.

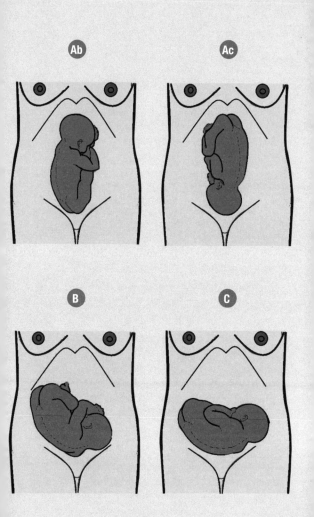

The A to Z of the Reproductive and Sexual Organs

Bladder

Macroscopic view
Coronal - Male

The male bladder is on the prostate gland, which if it hypertrophies crushes the urethra & hence affects urine & the ejaculate. Excessive filling will cause retrograde flow and affect the kidneys. Pelvic injury can easily cause damage to the urinary bladder particularly if it is full at the time and rupture may cause peritonitis due to infected urine in the pelvis.

1 parietal peritoneum
2 Ileum
3 paravesicular space
4 ureteric orifice (opening of the ureter) - in the bladder trigone
5 Levator Ani m
6 Ischiopubic ramus
7 ischiorectal fossa - anterior recess
8 superficial fascia (Colles' fascia) + subcutaneous fat
9 vesical venous plexus
10 deep transverse peroneal muscle & investing fascia + adherent superficial peroneal fascia
11 corpus spongiosum (bulb of the penis)
12 urethra - with surrounding muscular sphincter - urethral sphincter
13 deep fascia of the penis AKA Buck's fascia
14 Ischiocavernosus m (lat) + Bulbocavernosus m
15 Corpus cavernosum m
16 Obturator internus m + investing fascia
17 pelvic fascia AKA endopelvic fascia
18 internal urethral orifice
19 vesicular fascia
20 Detrusor m - smooth muscle wall of the bladder
21 internal vesicular mucosa - lining transitional epithelium

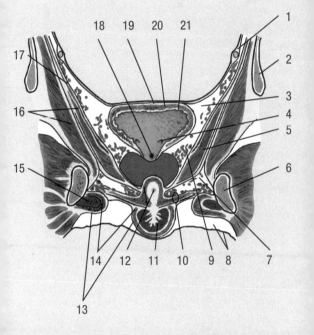

Bladder

Macroscopic view

Parasagittal - looking in from the side - Male

The male bladder is closely associated to all the other pelvic structures, particularly the prostate; each with separate fascial coverings, but an anastomotic BS, and many well defined inter-organ spaces, (in order to facilitate the changing volumes passing through these areas). The extent of any cancer spread is affected by these factors - obstruction via the fascial coverings but blood born spread due to the copious BS located in the spaces b/n the organs.

1 visceral peritoneum
2 serosal layer adherent to the bladder AKA Tunica adventitia
3 ductus deferens
4 subcutaneous fat
5 Detrusor m - smooth muscle wall of the bladder AKA Tunica muscularis
6 Pubis
7 Corpus cavernosum
8 Corpus spongiosum
9 Glans penis + covering foreskin
10 Testis - covered by the scrotal sac (note the subcutaneous Dartos m)
11 Epididymus
12 retropubic space + pubovesicular m
13 Crus of the penis + urogenital diaphragm
14 Bulbospongiosus m covering the Bulb of the penis
15 Bulbourethral gland AKA Cowper's gland
16 Prostate gland + retroprostatic fascia AKA Donovillier's fascia
17 EAS + anus
18 Levator Ani m
19 presacral fascia
20 rectal fascia AKA Waldeyer's fascia
21 seminal vesicle
22 rectovesicular pouch
23 Sacrum
24 R ureter
25 sigmoid colon

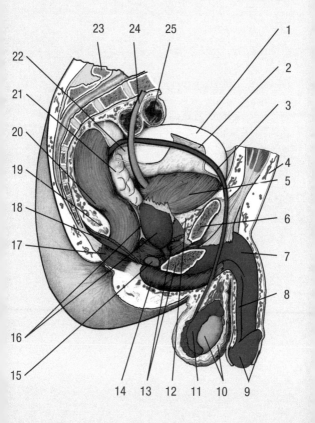

© A. L. Neill

Bladder

Macroscopic view
Lateral - male - BS

The bladder is a collapsible bag which has a copious anastomotic BS intimately related to the adjacent structures - prostate in the male - vagina and uterus in the female.

1   int. iliac a & v
2   obliterated umbilical a
3   superior vesical a
4   fundus
5   median umbilical lig
6   vesical venous plexus
7   prostate brs from inf. vesical a & v
8   prostate
9   urethra
10 seminal vesicles
11 middle rectal v
12 ductus deferens + a
13 ureter + uteric a + v
14 inf. vesical uteric a & v
15 inf. gluteal a & v

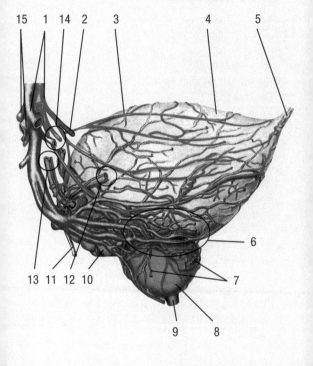

15   1   14   2   3   4   5

6

7

13   11   12   10

9   8

Breast

Macroscopic view

A   Anterior skin removed laterally

B   Parasagittal

The breast is a modified superficial sweat gland, situated b/n the skin and the deep fascia overlying the chest wall muscles.

1   muscles of the anterior chest wall
    i = intercostal m
    p = Pectoralis Major m

2   remnants of the deep fascia - overlying the muscles of the chest wall

3   glandular T of the breast (g) - arranged in lobes (L) & smaller lobules

4   subcut. fat - b/n the skin & deep fascia

5   tubercles of the areolar glands

6   nipple = papilla of the mammary gland

7   areola - pigmented T surrounding the nipple

8   lactiferous
    d = ducts - opening into larger sinuses
    s = sinuses in the areolar region

9   skin - with CT septa extending into the fat through to the deep fascia - they act as supportive bands for the breast T & if they extend into the axilla are called Copper's ligaments (not shown)

10   intermammillary sulcus

11   Clavicle

12   ribs
    i = first rib
    ii = second rib

13   intercostal muscles - intercostal BVs & Ns lie in b/n

14   lung T & pleural lining

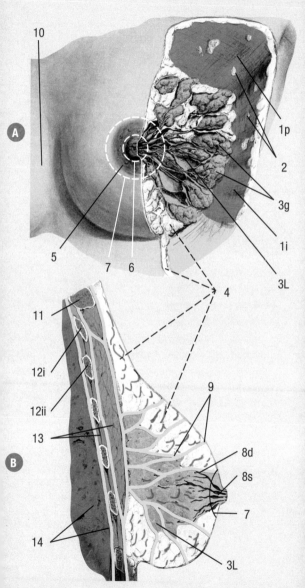

A

10

1p

2

3g

1i

3L

5

7 6

4

B

11

12i

12ii

13

9

8d

8s

7

14

3L

© A. L. Neill

Breast

Histology
LP & HP H&E glandular changes

A *Mature*
B *Early pregnancy*
C *Late pregnancy*
D *Lactating*

The breast is one of the body's exocrine glands which undergo radical changes in life, from infancy to puberty, maturity - to pregnancy, lactation and menopause. It is strongly influenced by Hs which determine its size, shape and function.

The adipose & glandular T ↑ with maturity and during pregnancy & particularly in lactation, replacing the fibrous CT which returns in menopause.

1 lobe of glandular T
2 CT b/n lobules - interlobular CT
3 CT w/n lobules - intralobular CT
4 intralobular ducts
5 interlobular ducts (excretory)
6 adipose cells
7 myoepithelial cells - outside the ducts to compress them
8 alveoli
9 lactiferous ducts
10 BVs
11 apocrine cells (& holocrine)
12 secretion with portions of the secreting cells & vacuoles

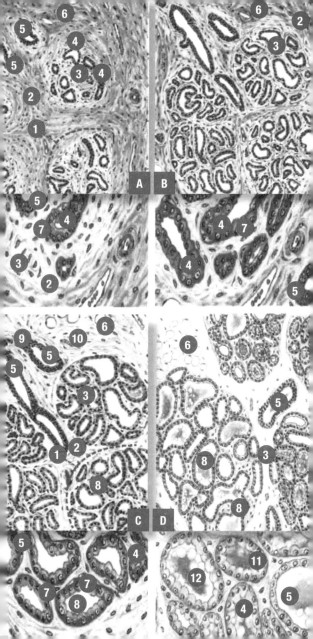

Breast AKA Mammary gland
Cell types

mammary gland cell
Schema HP

The breast is composed of fibroconnective tissue interspersed with glands which change with the menstral cycle, pregnancy & menopause. The glandular cells secrete protein granules via pinocytotic vesicles & fat droplets into the acinar lumen (along with some cytoplasm & vesicles) & then ducts compressed by the surrounding myoepithelial cells.

1   fat droplet
2   cytoplasmic rim
3   protein granule secretion
4   pinocytic vesicle = protein
5   mitochondria
6   GA
7   nucleus
>   m = nuclear membrane
8   lysosomes
9   ER
>   S = smooth ER
>   R = rough ER (ribosomes attached)
10 BM
11 myoepithelial cell process
12 nucleolus
13 mv

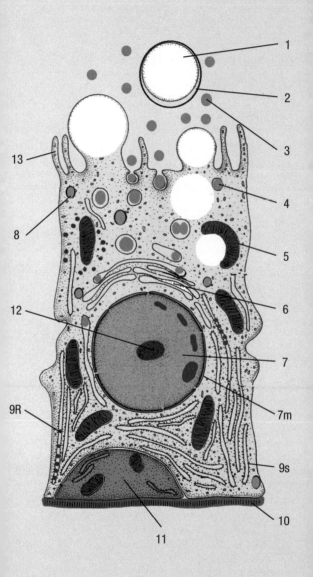

81

Breast

Blood Supply - arterial

1 thoracoacromial a
2 pectoral br
3 lateral thoracic a
4 subscapular a
5 posterior intercostal a
6 perforating br
7 lateral mammary br
8 thoracodorsal a
9 internal thoracic a

      a = anterior intercostal br
      m = medial mammary br
      p = perforating br

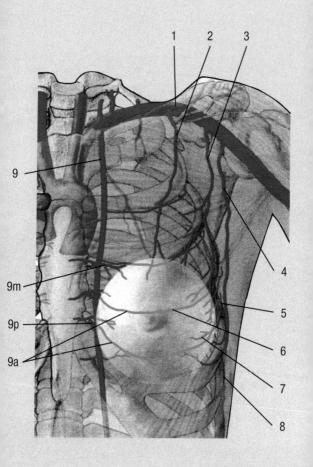

Breast

Blood Supply - venous & LNs

The breast drains mainly to the 40 axillary LNs from 3 levels. Using Pectoralis Minor m as a guide these can be described as those lateral to Pec. Minor (3, 4, 6 & 9), medial to Pec. Minor (15 &18) & below Pec Minor (2 & 16), but the only palpable LNs are : the anterior & central LNs in the axilla and the supraclavicular LNs.

The venous supply mirrors the arterial supply and LNs flank the veins.

In breast cancer the number of axillary LNs involved is correlated to the number of axillary LNs involved - in both male & females, with particularly poor survival associated with supraclavicular LN involvement.

1   axillary v
2   central LNs
3   lateral LNs AKA Humeral LNs
4   subscapular LNs
5   subscapular v
6   pectoral LNs (Sorguis' LN)
7   lateral thoracic v
8   thoracodorsal v
9   paramammary LNs
10 superior lat quadrant
11 inferior lat quadrant
12 inferior medial quadrant
13 internal thoracic v
14 superior medial quadrant
15 parasternal LNs
16 interpectoral LNs (Rotter's LNs)
17 Pectoralis minor m
18 apical LNs
19 supraclavicular LNs (Virchow's LNs)

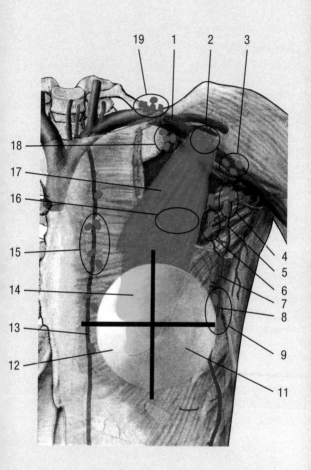

Breast
Stages of development

Macroscopic view

The breast is a modified superficial sweat gland, situated b/n the skin and the deep fascia overlying the chest wall muscles. It has 5 stages of development. Thelarche (2) or breast budding is the first sign followed by pubarche AKA adrenarche (3) the appearance of pubic hairs & the rapid breast growth along with the menarche (4) (the onset of menstruation). Breast development may be asymmetrical initially but in most cases this is regularized, by the time of the maturation of the breast and development of the adult pattern of pubic hairs (5). Any sign of breast development before 8yo in girls is considered precocious puberty, and often related to the weight of the child &/or ethnic origin.

1 Pre-adolescent - elevation of the papilla alone
2 Breast bud stage -elevation of the breast & papilla (9-10yo)
3 Further enlargement of the breast T w/o separation & the appearance of pubic hairs (10-11yo)
4 Projection of the areola & papilla forming a $2°$ mound above the breast (12-14yo)
5 Mature stage - projection of the papilla alone (14-16yo)

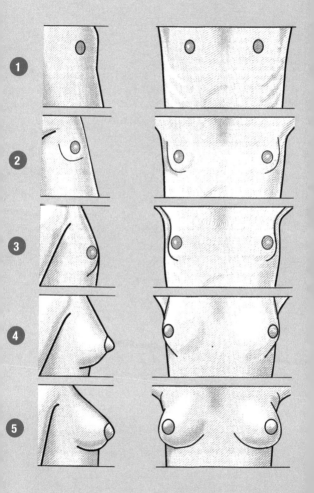

Breast
Stages of development

Functional changes
Schema

The breast has 3 functional changes. Initial rudimentary glandular formation; growth & glandular development in pregnancy; lactation for breast feeding. After which the glands will regress but remain present until the menopause when most of the T will be replaced with fat & fibrous T.

1 **mature breast - rudimentary glandular development, with adipose T, (a) fibroconnective T (f) and rudimentary glands (g) & ducts (d)**
2 **pregnant breast stimulated by the ovary & placenta showing rapid gland growth (g) with fibrous septa (f)**
3 **lactating breast enlarged with tortuous glands (g) filled with secretions**

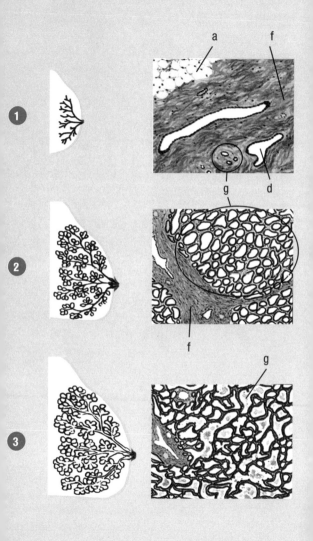

Breast Examination (BE)

Observation

Monthly self breast examination (SBE) is recommended for women, and biannual SBE for men. Any changes should be reported to a medical professional.

SBE starts with observation. Standing in front of the mirror, with arms at the sides - inspect the breasts looking for any changes, noting the area of the breast.

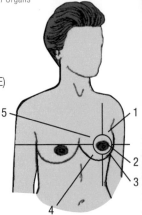

Changing posture such as: placing the hands on the hips, head or tensing the chest wall muscles will emphasize any changes.

1   upper outer quadrant
2   central area - includes the nipple & areolar area
3   lower outer quadrant
4   inner lower quadrant
5   upper inner quadrant

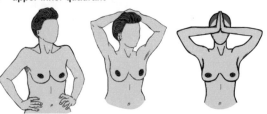

Changes looked for in particular are the following:

A   changes in size & shape of the breasts
B   a rash or redness on the skin &/or around the nipple
C   nipple discharge (1 or both)
D   lump/swelling in the armpit (axillary LNs) or the Clavicle (Virchow's node)
E   lumps / thickenings in the breast outline
F   skin puckering / texture changes
G   nipple changes e.g. position, shape, inversion
H   pain in the breast &/or axilla

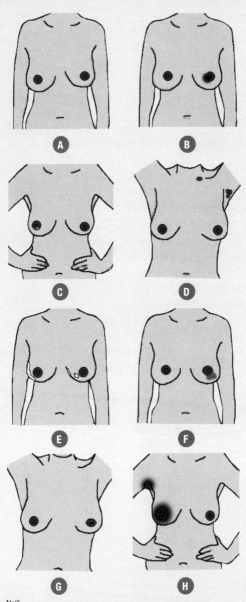

Breast Examination

Palpation

Palpation of the breast using one or both hands is the next step in breast examination.

Using the flat of the fingers (rather than the fingertips), the breast tissue is examined at 3 levels: light touch, medium touch & firm pressure.

Nipples are then individually examined for differences & squeezed if to illicit discharge if one is not observed - this is not necessary if the nipple is perceived to have changes when being observed, or the nipple/areolar is pierced.

1. palpation when standing up can be done in the shower - where there is less friction

   heavy or pendulous breasts may need to be supported with the other hand

2. palpation patterns

3. palpation when supine - may need to support heavy or pendulous breasts with the other hand

4. squeezing of the nipples to illicit a discharge, do not do this if the breast is painful or discharge has been observed - note if pierced there may be fibrosis in the nipple areolar area, which may feel hard & sclerotic

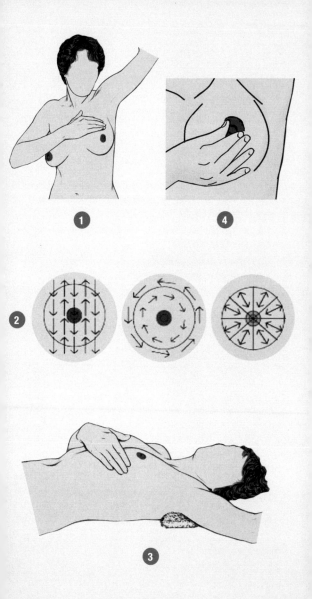

Breast

Lactation reflexes
A overview of the lactation reflexes
B HP view of the breast glandular tissue

During breast feeding the suckling o the baby stimulates 2 reflexes which effectively make the milk available, by: increasing milk production in the glandular cells (PROLACTIN) which swells the acini & squeezing milk from the glands into the ducts (OXYTOCIN).

1 suckling causing N impulses to go to the brain
2 via the hypothalamus → posterior pituitary gland → release of OXYTOCIN
3 via the hypothalamus → anterior pituitary gland → release of PROLACTIN
4 glandular complex made up of .....
5 myoepithelial cells surrounding the glandular acini contract around the glands forcing the contents into the ducts
6 glandular tissue

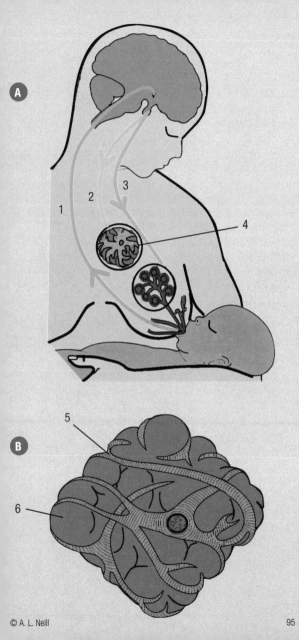

Breast

Morphological classification

The breasts, more than other organs change, often quite radically, with: age / lactation / hormonal & weight variations, and other body changes. So although there are features consistent with age changes, particularly menopausal changes, a better way to describe breasts is to consider their whole morphology, particularly as surgery on the breast is one of the commonest procedures for a number of reasons - one of the major reasons being dissatisfaction with their size & shape.

1 Breast Separation defn: horizontal distance b/n 2 breasts at the centre of the chest

<u>Touching breasts</u> AKA Kissing breasts - when standing upright w/o a bra, the breast touch.	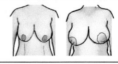
<u>Separate breasts</u> - commonest form of breast separation; 1 -2 finger breadths distance b/n breasts	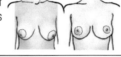
<u>Splayed breasts</u> separation b/n the breasts is wider inferiorly than it is superiorly (triangular shape b/n the breasts)	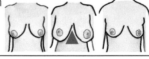
<u>Wide-set breasts</u> separation b/n the breasts is > 2 finger breadths	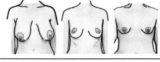
<u>Wide-set/ splayed breasts</u> - separation is > 3 finger breadths and is wider inferiorly than superiorly	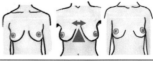
<u>Symmastia</u> - is the extreme of touching breasts. There is not any separation b/n the 2 breasts, and the tissue is full across the chest wall	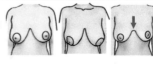

© A. L. Neill

2 Upper Breast fullness defn: the volume of the breast in the upper portion, this is the normal morphology of the younger breast & the "ideal" shape i.e. this is the shape of breasts with implants

<u>Full upper breast curve</u> convex line above the breast apex - with age; when there is weight loss &/or after breast feeding, the loss of this 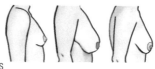 upper curve is the first change to occur in the breast shape. This is the ideal or standard shape of the younger breast.

<u>Semi full upper breast curve</u> - some fullness remains but the upper breast curve is not so convex - one of the first signs of normal breast aging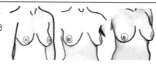

<u>Shallow upper breast curve</u> - the upper breast curve is straight or slightly concave - this may be a sign of age &/ or illness but many women develop with this shape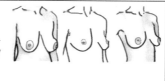

<u>Deflated upper breast curve</u> - loss of any upper fullness with the weight concentrated in the lower portion, which then tends to aggravate the situation & 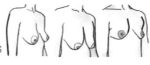 make the breasts sagging & pendulous, pulling them down. This can occur in large or small breasts & is aggravated by unsupported or poorly breasts when exercising particularly in high impact activities

<u>Oversized upper breast mass</u> - a convex upper breast curve with a down pointing breast apex (nipple). In this case the breast may appear deflated or masculine, when it is not.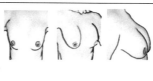

3 Breast Position defn: the position of the breast on the central chest, determined by the supportive ligaments in particular Cooper's lig. There is no way to alter the breast position as ligaments cannot contract but with agitation such as high impact sports activities, time & weight they will stretch.

<u>Self-supporting breasts</u> - the bottom of the breast in profile is perpendicular to the chest wall, & wearing a bra does not significantly alter the profile of 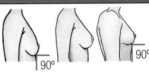 the upper breast curve. There is no breast crease. Note a breast may grow lower on the chest & appear "sagging" but the angle of the chest wall to the breast will reveal this is not the case

<u>Semi-supported breasts</u> - there is a clear breast crease (b) line on the chest where the breasts meet with the chest wall, only minimal changes can be seen when wearing a bra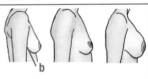

<u>Settled breasts</u> - while the nipple remains above or at the level of the breast crease, the main breast 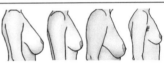 mass is below it. This is a further sign of aging in some women but it may also result from pregnancy ± breast feeding, weight loss, hormonal changes &/or severe illness.

<u>Pendulous breasts</u> - both the nipple and main breast mass are below the breast crease (b), with the nipple generally 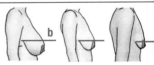 down pointing. This position is exacerbated by prolonged breast feeding or multiple pregnancies & extreme weight loss. While irreversible, it can be prevented from developing, by supporting the ligaments e.g. with a bra.

4 Breast Shape defn: the shape of the breast mass.

Archetype breast shape - AKA the standard breast shape. This is the ideal shape and most breast implants are modelled on this shape.

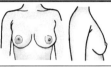

Uneven breast shape - this is very common if it is < 1 bra cup size (A); any larger & it is probably not just a normal variation in breast development (B) but due to other factors including an illness during breast development, asymmetrical activities in the upper torso - e.g. sport or occasionally this will occur with menopause

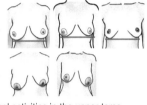

Conical breast shape - the breast is not round but cone shaped, it is generally a normal variant, particularly of small breasts.

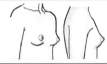

Thin breast shape - AKA tuberous breasts, the base of the breast is small causing it to protrude & appear smaller & thinner

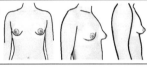

Omega breast shape - AKA a ball-shaped breast, a shape of mainly larger breast sizes, where the base is smaller than the widest circumference of the breast so the breasts can appear to be "kissing" & splayed. This is not a natural or common shape, & the breasts can appear disproportionably large for the body.

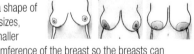

Reduced projection breast shape - the base circumference is too large for the breast mass. This also is not a natural or common shape but may be the result of breast reduction surgery, a smaller breast on a bigger base, as seen in the profile showing the original breast outline before reduction.

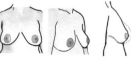

5 Breast Apex direction defn: the pointing of the breast - indicated by the pointing of the nipple.

<u>Forward pointing</u> - this is the standard position. This is the ideal shape and most breast implants are modelled on this shape.

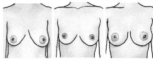

<u>Outward pointing</u> - this is also very common, and is often associated with the splayed ± wide breast separation.

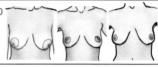

<u>Downward pointing</u> - associated with pendulous breasts & deflated breast curve

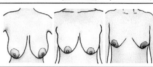

<u>Upward pointing</u> - this is only seen in deflated breasts

6 Nipple + Areolar size & shape

<u>Prominent erect nipples</u> - nipples may be erect, flat or inverted. Any changes not explained by events such as lactating or hormonal changes, may be considered important, & need to be investigated in case they signify occult disease processes including cancer. This is particularly significant if the changes are asymmetrical (e.g. one nipple becomes inverted) or there are associated skin changes. After lactation, the size and presentation of the nipples may change

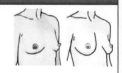

<u>Large areolars</u> - the size colour & shape of the areolar can vary considerably, from non-pigmented to deeply darkened, and b/n 1cm -8cm in diameter. They are generally circular but with erect nipples or after lactation may become oval.

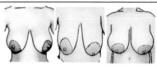

7 Chest morphology - influence on the breast: the shape of the underlying chest wall - influences the breast

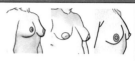

Pectus carinatum AKA barrel chest, when the breast bone (Sternum) is prominent means the breasts will appear widely spaced & splayed with an outward apex. This occurs naturally or with an overdeveloped diaphragm in athletes & singers.

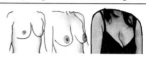

Pectus excavatum AKA hollow chested, when the breast bone (Sternum) is recessed, where the breasts will appear touching & possibly with a down pointing apex

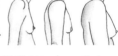

Scoliosis AKA spinal curvature present in 2% of women - this also occurs with poor posture e.g. round shoulders. The upper breast curve is flattened & the apex downward pointing, with the breasts appearing settled when they are self supporting

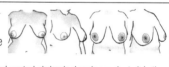

Distended epigastric region - AKA fat, high "stomach' - this is a common body shape in short stocky women &/or the overweight. The distended central abdominal region projects b/n the breasts, as a fatty pillow, making the breasts appear splay & or widely spaced.

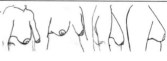

Excess skin in axilla region - with the arms at rest there appears to be a flap of skin on the side parallel to the floor. This is very common in those who have lost a great deal of weight, or the elderly woman. The breast is deflated and pendulous with associated skin creases in the axilla area, making it difficult to define the actual breast area.

Broad ligament

Macroscopic view
Posterior looking onto the uterus from behind

The uterus is extra peritoneal unlike the ovaries. The peritoneum covers it, folding over its anterior & posterior surfaces, forming pouches b/n the uterus and the bladder anteriorly & the rectum posteriorly. Pus, infection & endometrioses may be found in these dependant tissue pockets.

1. infundibulopelvic lig AKA suspensory lig of the ovary
2. ovary - which lies in the abdomen
   f = free margin - in the abodmen
   L = lateral margin
   m = medial margin
3. R ureter - w/n the 2 layers of the broad lig
4. extraperitoneal space
5. broad lig ant. & post. folds AKA mesometrium
   f = post. fold turns up to cover the ant. wall of the rectum
6. cervix - ant. & post labia present only in the parous woman
7. vagina
   a = anterior wall
   f = lateral fornix
   p = posterior wall note the rugae AKA horizontal folds on the surface
8. external os of the cervix (AKA orifice)
9. mesosalpinx
10. pivot of rotation & uterine movement
11. fimbria of ovarian tube
12. abdominal orifice of the infundibulum
13. ampulla of the ovarian tube
14. isthmus of the ovarian tube
15. fundus of the uterus
16. ovarian lig
17. ureter

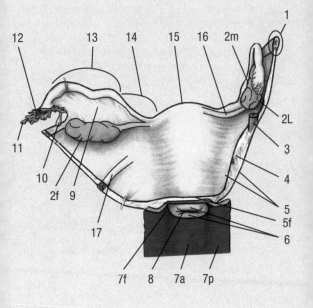

Bulbourethral glands AKA Cowper's glands

Macroscopic view
Coronal section with anterior tissue removed

The bulbourethral glands are the size of a pea located in the deep perineal pouch. These exocrine glands are at the base of the penis, lateral & posterior to the urethra. Their ducts are 2.5cm & pass through the perineal membrane and into the proximal portion of the spongy urethra. During SA, the glands produce the pre-ejaculate; a clear, viscous, salty fluid, which neutralizes the urethra & helps with lubrication. The female equivalent are the Skene's glands which can secrete 1-2 mls of clear fluid in the aroused female.

1. ureteral meatus - one point of the bladder trigone
2. muscular wall of the bladder AKA Detrusor m
3. internal urethral orifice
4. prostate gland + openings into the urethra
5. colliculus
6. opening of the utricle (male equiv of the uterus)
7. ejaculatory openings
8. urethral eminence in the membranous urethra
9. urogenital diaphragm containing Transverse peronei m
10. bulbourethral glands
    - o = openings in the urethra source of the pre-ejaculate
11. crus of corpus carvernosum
12. leading onto the shaft of the penis
13. cavernous urethra

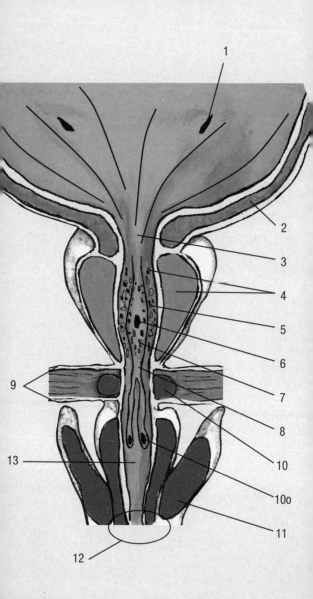

1

2

3

4

5

6

7

8

9

10

10o

11

12

13

© A. L. Neill

Bulbourethral glands AKA Cowper's glands

Histology
H&E showing gland structure & muscular capsule

The bulbourethral glands are a pair of small pea-shaped glands in the deep perineal pouch in the male. They are the equivalent of Bartholin's glands in the female. They diminish with age and are primarily simple exocrine tubuloacinar glands with a single opening into the urethra. They are surrounded by the sphincter urethrae. In arousal they secrete a material - the pre-ejaculate, which helps to lubricate the spermatic urethrae and facilitate the passage of the sperm in the ejaculate.

1 tubular part of the gland lined with columnar epithelium
2 skeletal m
3 collecting duct
4 acini
5 a & v in CT septum
6 CT septum

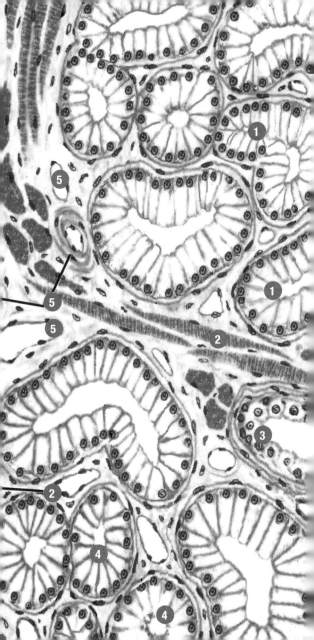

Cervix AKA Uterine Cervix

Histology –
LP overview H&E - oblique sagittal cut

The cervix is the firm fibrous neck of the uterus neck of the uterus, approx. 2-3cm in length - elongating in pregnancy. It protrudes into the vagina and is covered by the ectocervix - a non-keratinized stratified epithelium which is continuous with that of the lining of the vagina. The opening - external os - is continuous with the uterine cavity, lined by the columnar epithelial cells & mucoid glands - endocervix. The sperm must pass through the cervix to reach the uterine cavity & ovum. Muscle of the vaginal wall and the myometrium are continuous with the muscularis of the cervix. The cervical glands contribute to the vaginal lubrication, and assist the passage of the sperm.

1 muscularis = smooth muscle in the cervix
2 vaginal fornix
3 vaginal wall
4 venule
5 lymph nodule
6 mucous gland
7 vaginal cavity
8 transitional zone
9 external os - cervical canal
10 ectoderm = stratified non-keratinized epithelium
11 endoderm = simple columnar epithelium
12 cervical cyst
13 lamina propria

Note - cervical smears are taken at the sites of 2, 8, & 10 at least.

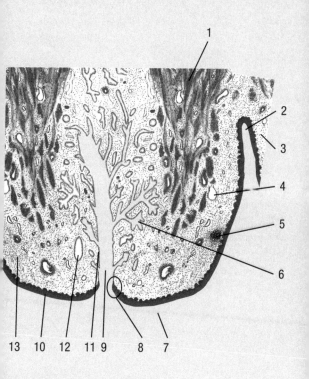

Clitoris

Macroscopic view

A   Anterior view - in situ

B   Anterior view with the surface vulval tissue removed

The clitoris is the female equivalent of the penis complete with all its equivalent parts & the same BS & NS similar number of nerve endings & sensitivity.

1   hood & shaft of the clitoris (equiv of the foreskin of the & shaft of the penis) + connecting frenulum

2   glans of the clitoris (equiv of the glans penis)

3   crus of the clitoris (covered by the corpus cavernosum m)

4   bulb of the clitoris (or vestibule)

5   external urethral meatus

6   vaginal opening

7   fossa navicularis = frenulum of the labia minora

8   labia minora

9   labia majora

10 anal opening

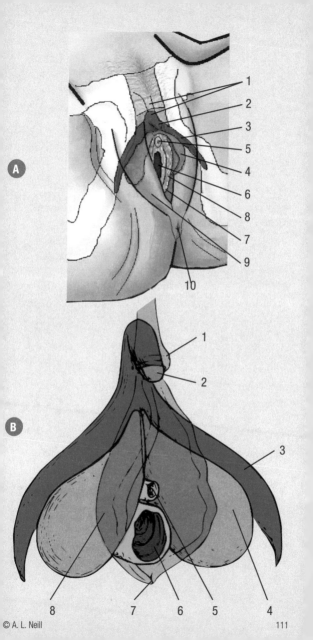

Cystocele AKA Bladder prolapse

Macroscopic view

A   Sagittal view

B   Anterior view

A cystocele is a displacement of the bladder wall into the vagina due to weakness caused by increased abdominal P which may be due to childbirth, straining &/or lifting heavy weights, along with being overweight & menopausal. It may also occur with other prolapses e.g. the uterine, rectal or intestinal.

Stage 1 protrudes into the vagina; Stage 2 visible at the vaginal introitus & Stage 3 protrudes through the vagina.

Symptoms include: urinary incontinence, inability to completely empty the bladder; recurrent UTIs; difficulty holding any intra-vaginal object in place e.g. a tampon; difficulty in starting, stopping or continuing to urinate, and a sensation of fullness or pressure inside the vagina.

1   peritoneal cavity
2   bladder
3   urethral sphincter
4   clitoris
5   urethral orifice
6   cystocele
7   anal opening
8   vestibule
9   external anal sphincter
10 rectum
11 uterus
12 openings of the ureter

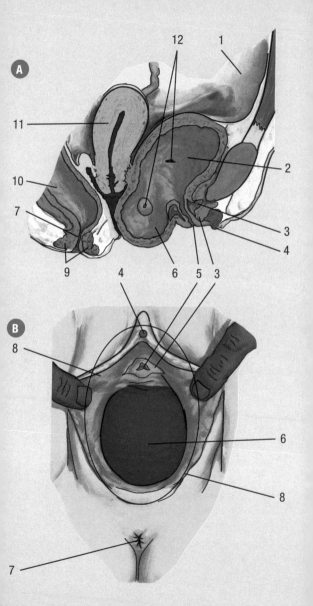

Ectopic pregnancies AKA Extra-uterine implantation

Schema

Ectopic pregnancies are any which occur outside the uterus. Predisposing factors are: previous ectopic pregnancies or previous abdominal or pelvic surgery including appendectomy; IVF Tx; IUCD in situ or PID

The commonest site of ectopic pregnancies are tubal implantation >98%.

Sites of implantation and their prevalence are broken down as follows

1. uterine ectopics = 2%
   - i = interstitial segment = 1.5%
   - c = cervical = .5%
2. isthmus of the oviduct = 25%
3. ampulla of the oviduct = 55%
4. infundibulum - fimbriated edge = 17%
5. abdominal cavity = .1%
6. ovary = .5%

please note that in regions 3 & 4 the oöcyte has a surrounding shell of follicular cells - the oocyte-cumulus complex which is shed during 3 - the highest % of ectopic implantation.

Ectopic - Tubal Implantation (TI)

7. TI
8. rupturing TI
9. absorption w/o extrusion
10. absorption with extrusion
11. intraperioneal ruptured TI with haematocele
12. ruptured TI into the Broad lig
13. incomplete TI
14. tubal blood mole

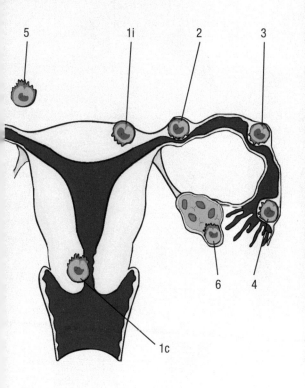

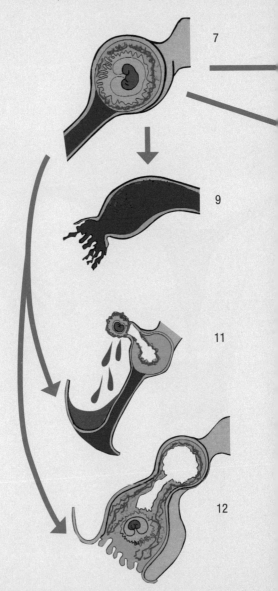

© A. L. Ne

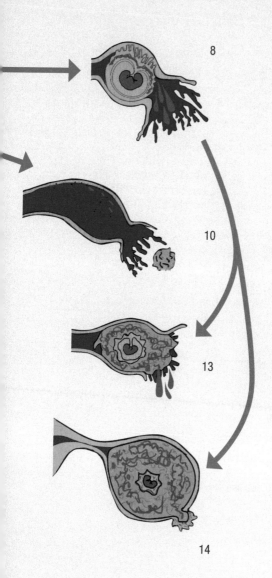

8

10

13

14

Ductus Deferens AKA Vas Deferens (VD)

Schema showing the sites & and procedure of a vasectomy

The ductus deferens carries the sperm from the testes, epididymis to the seminal vesicles where they are stored until ejaculation. When ejaculating they leave the seminal vesicles, pass through the prostate via the urethra. The prostate adds secretions to the sperm to help with their passage and preservation. The sperm leave the body via the penis. If any parts of this pathway ie blocked or cut, the ejaculate is rendered sterile. A vasectomy is the cutting (& possibly removing a section) of the VD. At least 2 -3 months must pass for all the sperm stored in the seminal vesicles are removed. Secondary blockages may develop after a vasectomy & the procedure cannot always be reversed as escaped sperm - leaving the cut end of the VD may cause the development of anti-sperm Abs, destroying the sperm in the testes.

1   ureter
2   bladder
3   ductus deferens AKA vas deferens
4   urethra (penile)
5   epididymis
6   testis
7   scrotum
8   pampiniform plexus
9   prostate
10 seminal vesicles

v   VASECTOMY LANDMARKS
   3v   division of theVD - may be a small cut or the removal of a section
   5v   site of secondary blockage after a vasectomy - preventing a successful reversal
   7v   site for the entry to cut the VD

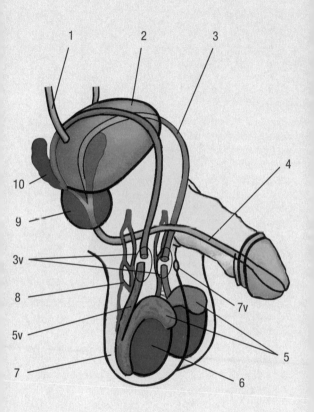

Endometriosis

A Schema - sagittal

B Macroscopic - sagittal view

C Microscopic view of the endometrial lining

D Macroscopic - superior view

E Macroscopic - deep internal view of the cervix

F Macroscopic - superficial view of the vulva

Endometriosis is ectopic endometrial tissue. It may be caused by retrograde flow of the menstrual tissue*, but this does not account for all the sites of endometriosis ie it may be found rarely in the eye. More than 40% of women have this ectopic tissue but with many it is destroyed by the resident macrophages. In 5-10% or women it persists, although this is only a rough approximation as unless the woman presents with symptoms that are then investigated endometriosis is not detected.

Infertility, pelvic pain, dysmenorrhoea, dyspareunia & menstrual irregularities are common presenting symptoms. Endometriosis is also found incidentally on laparoscopy.

commonest sites

1. bladder
2. pouch of Douglas (cul-de sac)
3. rectum
4. sacroiliac lig
5. broad lig
6. ovary

   c = ruptured ovarian / peritoneal cyst (AKA chocolate cyst)
7. sigmoid colon

rarer sites

8. umbilicus / site of laparoscopy
9. SI
10. appendix / LI
11. peritoneal cavity
12. round lig
13. perineal body / vulva
14. rectum
15. cervix

p = posterior fornix

other deposit sites

16. myometrium (with endometrial invasion is adenomyosis)
17. Bartholin's gland

* commonest sites follow a retrograde movement of the endometrial T and are marked with dark red circles ●

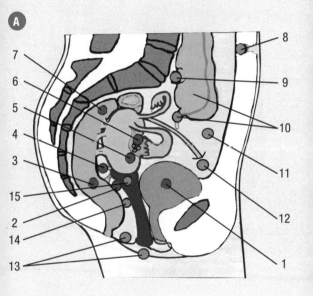

A

7

6

5

4

3

15

2

14

13

8

9

10

11

12

1

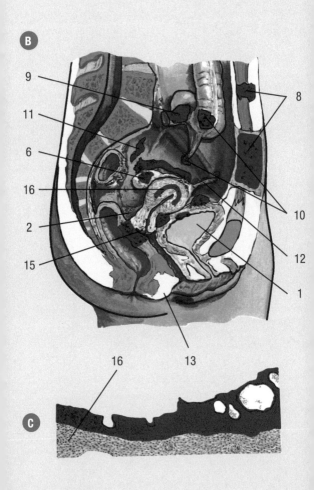

© A. L. Neil

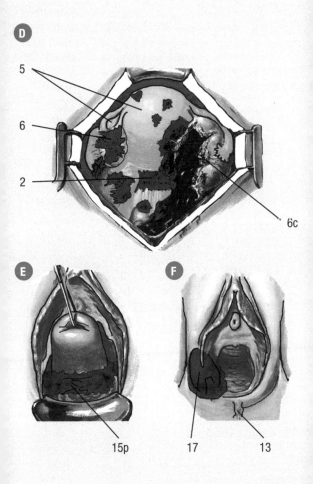

D

5

6

2

6c

E

15p

F

17 13

Erogenous zones

Schema

There is an extensive number of erogenous zones in the male & female, which vary in intensity. The following are guidelines as to the sites & intensities of each, as there is considerable individual variation. As a general principle it is better to begin with the less intense areas and move to those of greater intensity, rather than commence at those sites immediately.

	Site	Female	Male	Stimulation guide
1	Hair	++	++	Gentle
2	Ears	+++	+++	Moderate
3	Cheeks	++	+	Gentle
4	Lips / Kissing	+++++	++	Moderate
5	Neck - front & back (particularly at the hairline)	+++++	+++++	Moderate
6	Shoulders / UL	++	++	Gentle
7	Axilla / armpit	++	+++	Moderate
8	Breast Nipples	+++ +++++++	++ +++	Gentle Intense
9	Abdomen	++++	+++	Moderate
10	Naval	++++	+++	Moderate
11	Base of spine / lower back	++++	++++	Moderate
12	Buttocks	+++++++	+++++++	Intense
13	Genital area	+++++++++++	+++++++++++	Intense
14	Fingers / Toes			Intense - *as moderators or facilitators of arousal*
15	Insides of the thigh	+++++++	+++++++	Intense
16	Back of the knees	+++	+++	Moderate
17	Feet / soles	++++++	++++++	Moderate

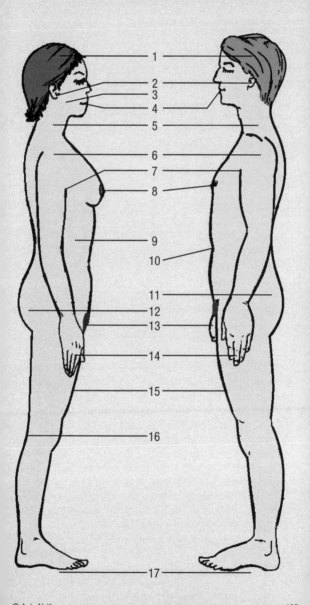

Erogenous zones - Female

Schema

Female erogenous zones are more widespread than those of the male, as is their degree of effectiveness.

1 **abdomen / umbilicus /**
gentle massage / circular motions / formation of pseudolabia with sides of the abdomen (for those with larger looser abdomens)

2 **axilla**
firm massage / oral caressing

3 **back - upper/lower**
light → firm touch & massage

4 **breasts / nipples - highly erogenous**
light → firm tactile stimulation / oral caressing / genital contact

5 **buttocks**
moderate → very firm touch & massage

6 **head / hair / face**
gentle tactile stimulation

7 **facial & cervical features in detail**
ear- earlobes / hairline / lips, mouth / neck
gentle tactile & oral caressing
note kissing can be more erotic than PV intercourse

8 **feet / soles / toes**
gentle → moderate tactile stimulation / oral caressing

9 **genital area**
including: anus clitoris, labia, mons pubis, perineal body, vaginal introitus & vestibule
a high variability of sensitivity corresponding to the large number of N endings in this area (the highest in the body in both male & female) mean that the effect of most forms of stimulation are amplified
tactile stimulation / oral caressing / genital contact

10 **inner thigh**
gentle → moderate tactile & oral caressing

11 **upper limb**
including shoulder / upper arm / forearm / hands (particularly palms) / fingers
light → firm touch & massage

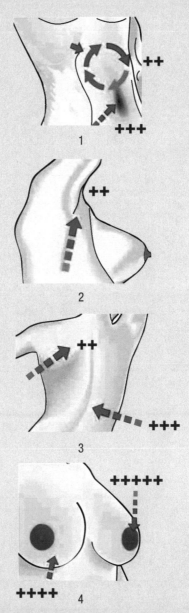

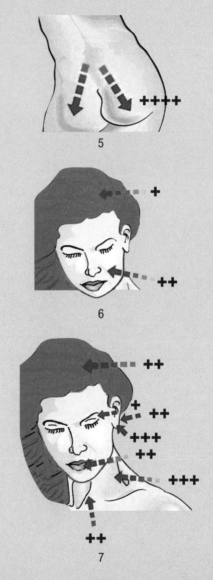

© A. L. Neil

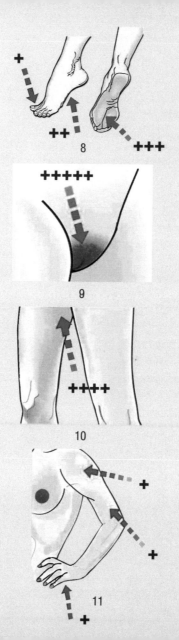

Fistulae

Macroscopic
Sagittal view
Parasagittal view

The fistulae are the abnormal passages b/n cavities. Because of the common walls shared by the crowded organs in the pelvic regions and diseases, which arise there, this area is particularly susceptible. These defects are very difficult to repair because of the friability of mm, and the Ps on the viscera. Consequences are socially difficult.

1 bladder
2 urethra
3 vagina
4 rectum
5 ureter (dilated)
6 uterus
7 broad lig
8 urethrovaginal fistula
9 vesicovaginal fistula
10 rectovaginal fistula
11 enterovaginal fistula
12 vesicocervical fistula
13 uretovaginal fistula

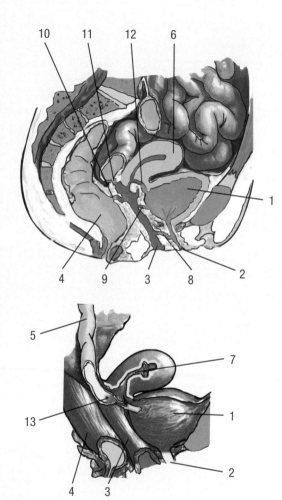

External genitalia - female

Macroscopic Anterior frontal view
Fascial support

The anterior abdominal wall holds the contents of the pelvis & abdomen in by a series of strong fascial sheets & ligaments. The external genitalia sit on the supportive fascia outside the peritoneum.

1 subcutaneous fat AKA Camper's fascia
2 deep fascial layer AKA Scarpa's fascia, which becomes more defined in the lower part of the abdomen
3 line where Scarpa's & Colle's fascia meet, separating 2 compartments & forming the inguinal lig -
4 ASIS
5 femoral a & v + N
6 cribiform fascia defect in …;
7 fascia lata (cut edge)
8 cloquet's (AKA Rosenmuller's) LN
9 deep femoral LN
10 ischiorectal fat deep to the skin
11 anus
12 Colle's fascia
13 saphenous vein
14 linea alba, CT line where the 2 sides of CT meet & attach

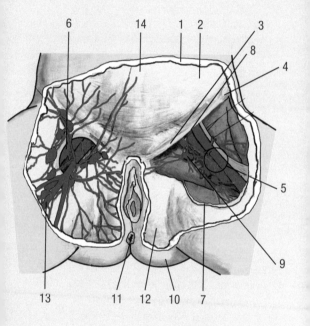

External genitalia - male

Macroscopic view
Anterior frontal fascial support

The deep fascia of this region (Colles' fascia) has several regional names. This layer is immediately deep to the superficial fascia (Camper's fascia). These layers maintain and separate the genitals from the peritoneum in the make, and are the main support of the pelvis and abdominal organs.

1   subcutaneous fat AKA Camper's fascia
2   deep fascial layer of the abdomen AKA Scarpa's fascia, which becomes more defined in the lower part of the abdomen merging with Colles's fascia along...13
3   fascia of the ext. oblique m
4   ASIS
5   femoral a & v
6   cribiform fascia defect in …;
7   fascia lata
8   internal spermatic fascia AKA Buck's fascia
9   ischeal tuberosity
10 ischiorectal fat - semi liquid in life
11 anus
12 Colle's fascia AKA deep fascial layer
      a = of the perineum
      b = of the scrotum AKA Dartos fascia
      c = of the penis AKA Dartos fascia
13 inguinal lig - separates the abdomen from the LL & perineum
14 saphenous vein
15 linea alba, CT line where the 2 sides of CT meet & attach

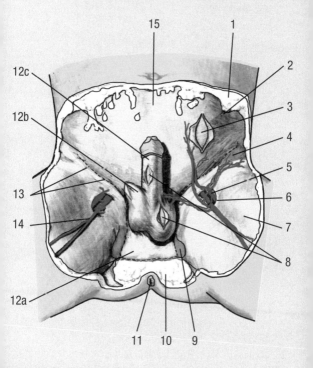

15

1

12c

2

3

12b

4

5

13

6

14

7

8

12a

11 10 9

Hymen

Macroscopic view

Inferior looking up into the Vestibule & Vagina

A   Annular hymen

B   Cribiform hymen

C   Septate hymen

D   Parous hymen

The hymen is a membrane which surrounds & partially closes the vaginal opening. It forms part of the vestibule & external genitalia, and is similar in structure to the vagina. In children it is thick & inelastic but with puberty thins to become discontinuous semitranslucent & elastic. The opening allows for the drainage of menstral blood, and is usually annular but may take other forms. Rarely it is imperforate and remains thickened. This requires an operation - hysterotomy. The effects of sexual intercourse and childbirth generally result in the destruction of the hymen leaving only remnants - caruncae myrtiformes. This may also result from disease, injury, medical examination, masturbation or even physical exercise. The measure of the hymen opening is performed by the insertion of a glass or plastic rod of 6mm diameter having a globe on one end with varying diameter from one to two and a half cm, the Glaister Keen rod. An intact hymen is not evidence of virginity nor is the absence of the membrane.

A truly imperforate hymen must be opened to allow for the release of menstral blood, or it may result in an haematocele.

1   hood of = prepuce of the clitoris (equivalent of the foreskin if the penis)

2   glans of the clitoris (equivalent to the glans of the penis)

3   labia minoris - inner lips, these may be larger and protrude outside of the outer lips

4   vaginal introitus

5   fossa navicularis

6   external urethral meatus

7   fibrous septate- which if very strong needs to be surgically divided

8   caruncae myrtiformes

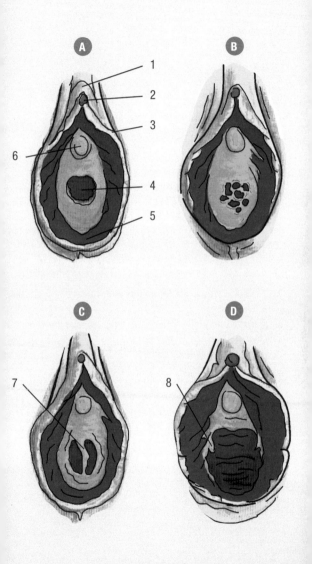

Hymen
Imperforate

Macroscopic view

A Inferior – looking onto the inferior surface of the imperforate hymen

B Sagittal – looking into haematocolpos

C Inferior – opening of the hymen to release contents

The hymen is a membrane which surrounds & closes the vaginal opening. It is similar in structure to the vagina. In children it is thick & inelastic. Rarely this continues into puberty, and may block or impede menstral bleeding causing build up in the vagina & eventually the uterus, of menstral & other discharge, leading to a haematocolpos. Depending upon the hymen, cutting in a cross to release the contents may suffice but often hysterotomy, i.e. complete removal of the hymen is needed, particularly if in association with infundibulation. Once opened it is important to prevent repair which re-closes the hymen.

1 hood of = prepuce of the clitoris (equivalent of the foreskin if the penis)
2 glans of the clitoris (equivalent to the glans of the penis)
3 labia minoris - inner lips, these may be larger and protrude outside of the outer lips
4 vagina
    i = introitus
5 hymen
6 cruciate cut
7 uterus
8 bladder – distorted by the blood – haematocolpos
9 rectum – distorted by the vaginal mass of blood and other contents

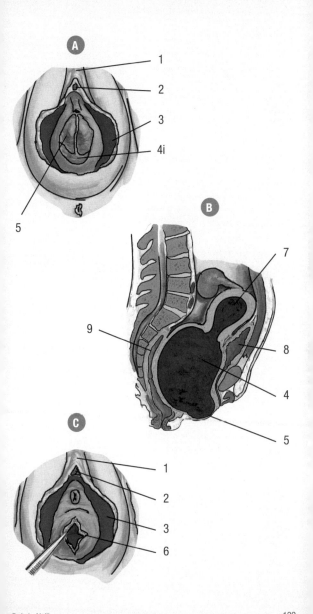

Hysterectomy

A *Macroscopic Superior view, - looking down onto the pelvis*

B *Schema of removal abdominally (B1) or vaginally (B2)**

C *Schema of contents removed in subtotal (i) total (ii) & radical (iii) operations*

Hysterectomy is the removal of the uterus. It is often associated with the removal of other related structures such as the cervix & ovaries. In this case these structures have also been removed.

1 bladder covered via the peritoneum
2 vagina
3 round lig
4 obturator LN
5 uterine BVs - ligated
6 external iliac LNs
7 hypogastric LN
8 infundibulopelvic lig AKA suspensory lig
9 sigmoid colon
10 pouch of Douglas
11 uterosacral lig - ligated
12 obturator N
13 broad lig
14 ureter

* Removal via the vagina may place a strain on the supporting ligs & damage the adjacent structures and lead to prolapse of the bladder &/or rectal wall, now that it is not protected by the presence of the uterus.

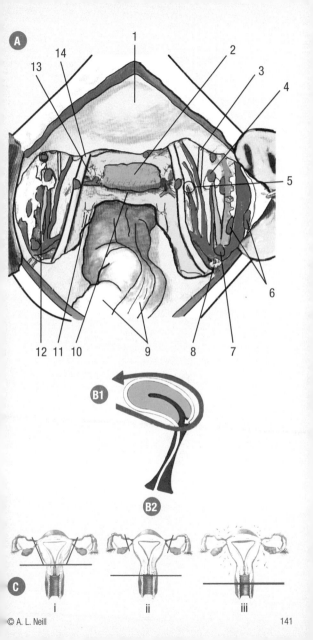

Implantation
Oöcyte to Blastocyst

Schema

The oöcyte is released from the mature follicle protected by the corona radiata - a crown of follicular granulosa cells, which fall off in the next 2-3 days as the egg moves along the fallopian tubes. Towards the end of the ampulla the sperm penetrates the protective ZP & fertilizes the ovum, after which no other sperm can enter the cell.

1 Day 1 after fertilization the egg cleaves forming 2 cells w/n the ZP & extruding the 2 polar bodies (1p)
2 Day 2 further cleavage forms the 4 cell stage
3 Day 3 it has continued to divide evenly producing more but smaller & smaller cells
4 Day 4 at approximately 32 cells the structure is now a Morula - a solid group of similar cells - the last stage before polarization develops
5 Day 5 the Blastocyst forms - cells divide into the inner cell mass, which becomes the embryo & the outer cell mass which becomes the placenta - and it implants into the uterine wall after dissolution of the ZP
6 uterus
7 ampulla of the fallopian tube - site of fertilization
8 mature ovum released from ...
9 the ovary

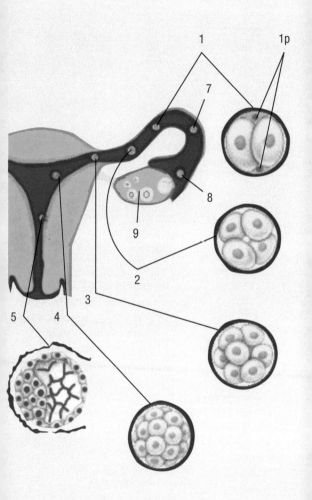

© A. L. Neill

143

Implantation
Blastocyst

Schema

A - sites of implantation in the uterus (a)

B - Day 4 dissolution of the ZP - to allow implantation

C - Day 5 beginning of implantation

D - Day 6-7 formation of the syncytiotrophoblast

E - Day 7-8 invasion beneath the uterine epithelium

F - Day 9 full implantation of the blastocyst, formation of amniotic cavity

G - Day 10 fibrin plug seals the blastocyst from the uterine cavity

H - Day 11 invasion of the endometrial capillaries into the syncytium

I - Day 12 formation of an internal syncytial arterial & venous flow

The Blastocyst implants into the uterine wall & invades the maternal capillaries & forms its own BS via a syncytium i.e. a multinucleic layer of cytoplasm. This becomes the placenta & the inner cell mass becomes the foetus & later the embryo.

1 ZP

2 inner cell mass - epiblasts

3 inner cell mass - hypoblasts

4 outer cell mass - cytotrophoblasts

5 blastocoele = Blastocyst cavity

6 uterine epithelium

7 BM

8 outer cell mass - syncytiotrophoblasts
   s = syncytium

9 uterine mucosa

10 amniotic cavity

11 maternal capillaries
    e = eroded capillaries by the syncytium

12 fibrin plug

13 growing hypoblasts - when they complete ventrally - formation of Heuser's membrane

14 syncytial lacunae

15 syncytial lacunae filled with blood - will become the BS of the placenta

16 extra-embryonic reticulum

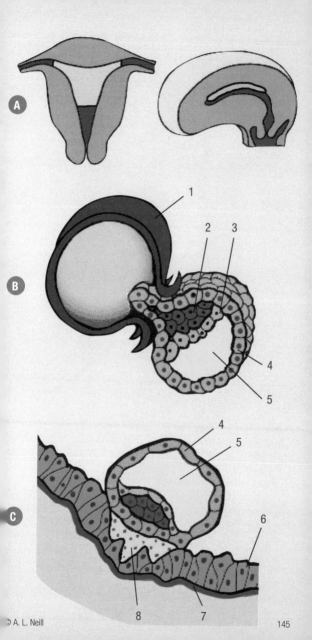

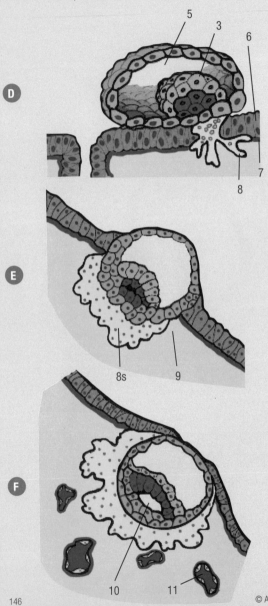

© A. L. Ne

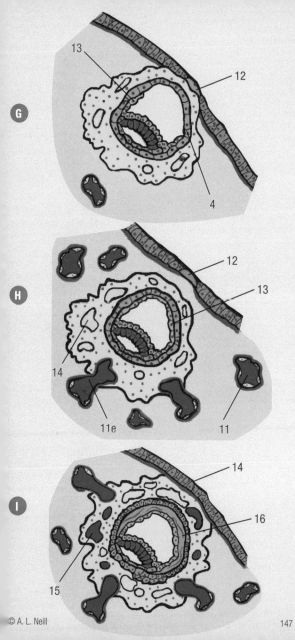

G

13

12

4

H

12

13

14

11e

11

I

14

16

15

© A. L. Neill

Meiosis

Schema

Most cells divide asexually - **mitosis** and are an exact replication of the original cell. These daughter cells have 2 sets of chromosomes, one from the father and one from the mother. **Sexual division AKA meiosis** reduces the cell's DNA from 2n = diploid to n = haploid. Hence when the 2 germ cell types ova - from the female & sperm from the male form the new zygote it will contain a set of chromosomes from each one. To remove the extra DNA in the female the ovum will form 2 polar bodies in their unequal divisions, leaving only 1 germ cell, the male will form 4 spermatozoa.

1 first polar body
2 second polar body
3 4 spermatozoa AKA sperm
4 ovum

MEIOSIS only - reduction division	
PROPHASE A	chromatin is duplicated and aligns itself into parallel sister chromosomes - and then the **chromatin is swapped from 1 gene to another changing the make up of each chromosome** otherwise the same as for mitosis
Meiosis / Mitosis	
METAPHASE B	chromosomes move along the microtubules to the centre of the cell
ANAPHASE C	chromosomes move to the opposite poles of the spindle & the cell elongates
TELOPHASE D	new NMs form chromatin detaches from the spindle
CYTOKINESIS E	new CMs form but **1 new cell is produced and 1 polar body (1) in the female (2n) 2 new cells in the male (2n)**
Meiotic reduction divisions	
PROPHASE A2 METAPHASE B2 ANAPHASE C2 TELOPHASE D2 CYTOKINESIS E2	The process is repeated w/o duplication to return reduce the cells to haploid so they can become full germ cells. **THE OVUM (n) in the female and the second polar body (2) 4 SPERMATOZOA (n) in the male**

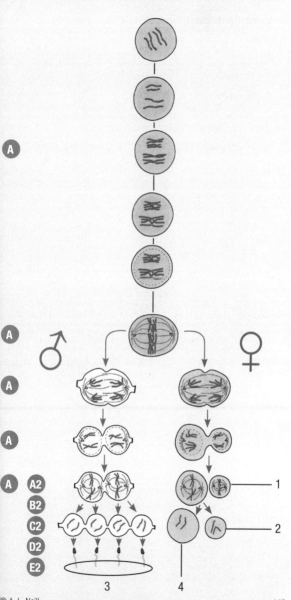

Menopause AKA Climateric

Schema

Menopause **(C)** is defined as the period after cessation of menstruation, when fertility **(A)** ceases. In the beginning this may be difficult to determine as periods may be irregular for several years before they completely cease due to fluctuating H levels particularly oestrogen **(O)** - progesterone **(P)** usually declines in more regular pattern. This is Perimenopause **(B)**, note pregnancy is possible in this time. Although the term menopause includes all time after menstral cessation, the term Post-menopause **(D)** has been used to describe the following years as changes continue to occur for years afterwards. Most changes can be explained by the irregularity and finally cessation of the ovarian Hs, but there is a great deal of individual variation.

	Peri-(B) → Menopause (C)	→ Postmenopause >5yrs (D)
1 **Cerebral**	Fatigue / sleep disturbance headaches / Irritability mood changes	Sleep restored Mood restored Headaches cease
2 **Hair**	Loses body & shine Pubic hair ↑ may change pattern	Scalp Hair ↓ Facial & body hair ↑ Pubic hair ↓ becomes thinner & finer
3 **Endocrine**	Hot flushes due to vaso-instability ↓ ovarian Hs ↑ FSH, cortisol	Hot flushes ↓ & cease
4 **mouth / teeth**	Gum disease ↑	Gums recede ↑ Teeth loosen ↑
5 **Breasts**	lose firmness & elasticity nipples flatten	This plateaus nipple size ↓
6 **Bones & joints**	density ↓ osteoporosis ↑ arthritis	This process continues osteoporosis ↑ ↑ affects the spine causing kyphosis & back pain
7 **Central fat & Body muscle mass**	Fat deposits in the trunk ↑ Muscle mass ↓	Both trends continue & may increase in heart rate
8 **Cardiovascular changes**	↑ cardiovascular disease / atherosclerosis ↑ BP ↑ PVD	These disease processes continue & may increase
9 **Skin**	↑ skin dryness & flaccidity ↑ rougher texture ↑ nail	Continues - collagen loss causes skin thinness ↑ fragility
10 **GIT changes**	Abdominal bloating / appetite & taste changes	incontinence ↑ due to loss of muscle tone & prolapse
11 Uterus	↓ size	↑ fibrous content
12 **Ovary**	Become erratic in their H output ↓ response to FSH	Cessation of any H production ↓ size & ↑ fibrous content
13 **Vagina / Vulva**	Changes in discharge	Cessation of lubrication - hence dryness, thinning vaginal walls & shrinking vulval content
14 **Urinary changes**	↑ incontinence	UTIs ↑ - due to vaginal changes ↑ stress incontinence due to loss of muscle tone & prolapse

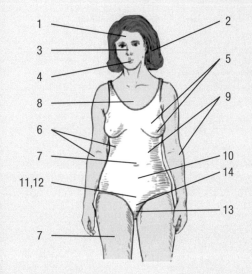

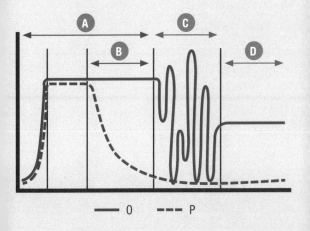

— 0   --- P

Menstruation
Endometrial changes - Shedding

Schema

The growing follicle initially produces oestrogen & after ovulation progesterone which stimulate the growth of the uterine wall vasculature. With the cessation of these Hormones after the loss of the unfertilized egg the uterine wall then starts to collapse and over a period of 3-8 days sheds 2/3 of its lining - containing b/n 10-80mls (average 30mls).

The endometrial menstral cycle is counted from the last day of menstruation i.e. the day bleeding ceases. Using a 28 day cycle as a model the stages of uterine wall changes are summarized below.

A   EARLY PROLIFERATION
Day 1-3 repair of the uterine wall is complete

B   PROLIFERATION (A + C)
Day 1-14 - uterine mucosa proliferates

C   LATE PROLIFERATION
Day 7-14 - growth of the uterine mucosa increases

D   LUTEAL PHASE
Day 14-20 - glands begin to coil & develop large secretory vacuoles & become tortuous

E   PREMENSTRAL PHASE
Day 20-23 -release of prostaglandins causes uterine cramping & local anoxia in the glands

F   MENSTRAL PHASE
Day 23-28 - dead and dying cells and glands begin to shed

1   endometrium = uterine mucosa
     b = basal
     s = superficial

2   plane of separation - top 2/3 of the uterine wall cleaved leaving the base below

3   myometrium = uterine muscular layer

4   uterine BVs

5   uterine glands & secretions

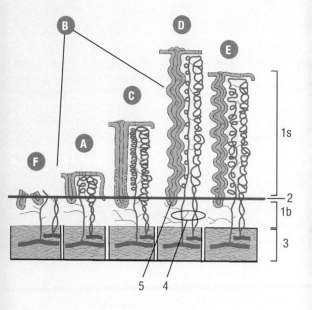

Menstruation
Hormone levels

Schema

The hypothalamus releases GNrH = GONADOTROPIN RELEASING HORMONE (i.e. a substance which allows for the secretion secondary substances which will cause the growth of follicles in the ovary) = 1

The anterior pituitary gland releases FSH = FOLLICLE STIMULATING HORMONE (i.e. a substance which stimulates the growth of follicles in the ovary) = 2

The anterior pituitary gland releases LH = LUTEINIZING HORMONE (i.e. a substance which stimulates the growth of the follicle in the ovary. It also causes ovulation - the release of an ovum from a mature follicle when it surges in the middle of the menstral cycle) = 3 *under the influence of the peak OE level.*

The ovarian follicle (FL) as it grows produces OE = OESTROGEN in increasing amounts, until ovulation = 4

The ovarian corpus luteum (CL) forms from the follicle after the release of the ovum. It continues to produce OE (4) at lower levels & starts to produce PR = PROGESTERONE = 5

The uterine wall grows thicker & more vascular under the influence of OE & PR

The hypothalamus stops producing GNrH (1) under the influence of OE & PR.

So the anterior pituitary stops producing FSH

The CL stops growing and stops producing OE & PR.

The uterine wall is no longer stimulated to grow and is shed.

The cycle begins again.

Day 1 is generally referred to as the beginning of the cycle, during the menstral or bleeding period.

Day 14 is generally the day of ovulation - mid cycle.

Most cycles are b/n 22 to 35 days, although there is considerable variation.

The cycle is divided into the FOLLICULAR PHASE (before ovulation) = F & the LUTEAL PHASE (after ovulation) = L. At ovulation (O) the egg/ovum is released and travels along the ovarian tubes to towards the uterus where it is usually shed.

F

0

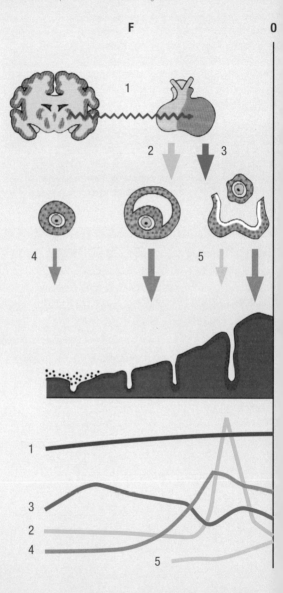

© A. L. Neill

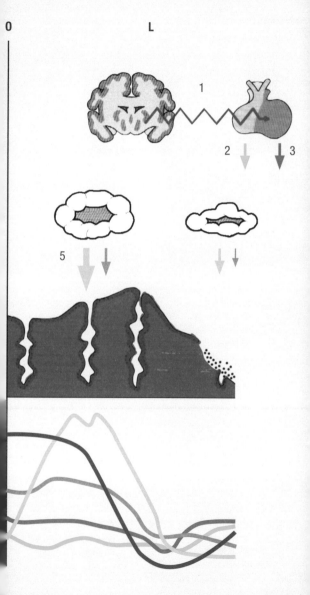

O   L

1

2   3

5

Breast - Nipple

Macroscopic view

A   nipple - sagital section / anterior view

B   inverted nipple

C   flat nipple

D   puffy nipple

E   normal nipple

The nipple is the outlet for the breast secretions, and there are 4 common types - **normal** - the nipple protrudes from the areola 1-2mm; **flat**, the nipple is level with the areola but can protrude when stimulated by sucking &/or temperature changes; **puffy** the nipple & areola T both are raised from the rest of the breast T & **inverted** - the nipple is adherent to the underlying T by strong bands of CT and points inwards.

Inverted nipples may prevent the milk from discharging causing it to build up beneath the areola, resulting in painful & swollen breasts and sore, cracked nipples.

1   skin
   a = areolar skin - pigmented, hairy (partic. at the outer edge) - it is the thinnest & most sensitive*
   b = breast skin - hairy, thin strong CT septa connect it to the underlying T
   n = nipple skin - pigmented - supported by conc. strong CT fibres attaching it to the subcutaneous T

2   lactiferous ducts

3   fibrous septa
   f = deep fibrous septa attaching the base to the deep fascia
   L = lobar & lobular septa dividing the glandular T
   n = attaching to the nipple
   s = supportive septa

   tethered to the skin - helps to maintain the breast shape & position - upper septa (AKA Cooper's lig) become stretched with age

4   lactiferous sinus - with surrounding smooth mu layers (outer circular & inner longitudinal) to help expel the glandular secretions

5   lactiferous duct openings

6   subcutaneous fat

7   glandular T - affected by Hs

8   increased subcut. fat of the breast T - also influenced by H levels

9   deep fascia overlaying the Pectoralis Major m

10 tubercles of areolar glands

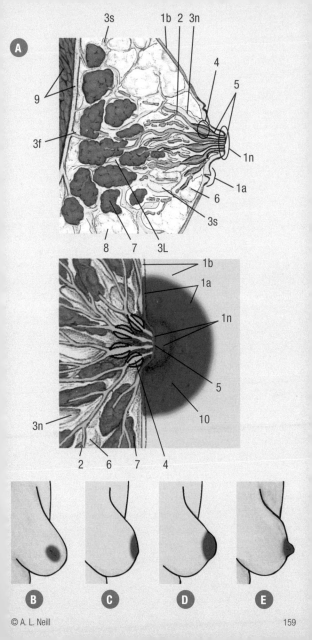

Breast - Nipple

Attachment - Feeding
Schema

A - baby attachment to the breast
B - nipple irritated by gums
C - nipple irritated by gums + tongue
D - ideal position gums on areola - nipple and areolar fully in the mouth

The baby needs to be able to "attach" to the nipple correctly in order to be able to suckle. This is generally with the nose touching the breast and the cheeks filling with the breast. Where the nipple is placed in the mouth is of great significance in the maintenance of breast feeding. The nipple is more sensitive than the areolar tissue, and chewing on it - impedes milk flow as the sinuses cannot empty efficiently, and causes cracked nipples.

1   areolar tissue
2   nipple
3   gums
4   tongue
5   lactiferous sinuses (in the areola)
6   palate

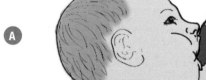

© A. L. Neill

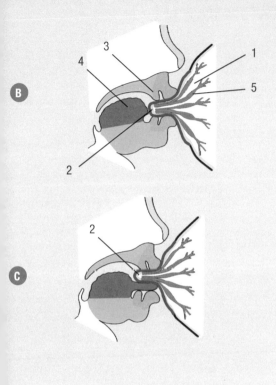

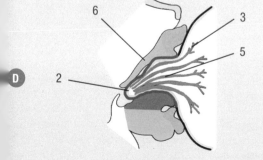

Oöcyte AKA Ovum AKA Egg

Schema HP
A = animal pole, V = vegetative pole
(polarity becomes more distinct with maturity)

The oöcyte is in the prophase of the first meiotic division in the primordial follicles and remains in this condition until there is further H stimulus. This spherical totipotent cell is one of the oldest in the body formed *in utero* & then laying dormant until stimulated at puberty by Hs. It is large varying from 50μm when immature to about 220μm at ovulation, just visible to the naked eye. Despite its shape it is polarized, & has a well developed CM, later forming the outer protective ZP. The eccentric nucleus has a prominent nucleolus & attached to it the Balbiani's vitelline body (BvB) which is crowded with concentrated organelles. The immature oöcyte is very active producing large amounts of protein, which diminishes with maturity, & is not restimulated again until fertilization. It is immobile & very sensitive to the environment, needing supportive cells to survive & generally only lives for 1-2 days after ovulation.

1. nucleus containing many pores partic around the BvB
2. compound aggregates - consisting of multiple vesicles, vacuoles & lipid droplets
3. mitochondria - concentrated in the BvB & dispersed throughout the cell
4. annulate lamellae
5. BvB - transient clustering of organelles
    t = transitional zone which is fibrous vesicular & contains ↑ SER (there is no membrane around the BvB)
6. cytocentrum - centre of the BvB filled with dense amorphous material, fibres & vesicles
7. GA - a number are dispersed throughout the cell & in the BvB
8. vesicles & vesicular complex in the BvB
9. wavy filaments
10. nucleolus
11. nuclear membrane - containing many pores partic around the BvB - used to facilitate communication b/n the nucleus & organelles
12. CM - note few mv - smooth featureless surface maximizing cytoplasmic volume

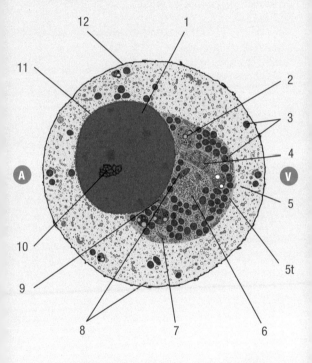

A

V

12

1

11

2

3

4

5

5t

10

9

8

7

6

Oöcyte-
Sperm penetration

Schema

The oöcyte when first released is protected by a crown of granulosa cells from the ovarian follicle. These cells slowly drop off as the ovum moves through the oviducts, leaving the bare ovum at the isthmus by which time a sperm has infiltrated the ovum. Once one sperm has entered the cytoplasm of the cell others are prevented from doing so by the release of the substances in the cortical granules.

1   nucleus
2   corona radiata - granulosa
     j = jelly coat
3   spermatozoa
     a = acrosomal ganule
     n = nucleus
     r = acrosomal reaction to push through the ZP
4   zona pellucida - protective covering of the ovum
5   CM + cortical granules
6   vitelline layer (outside CM)
7   1st polar body on the edge of the ovum - leaving the nucleus haploid
8   cytoplasm

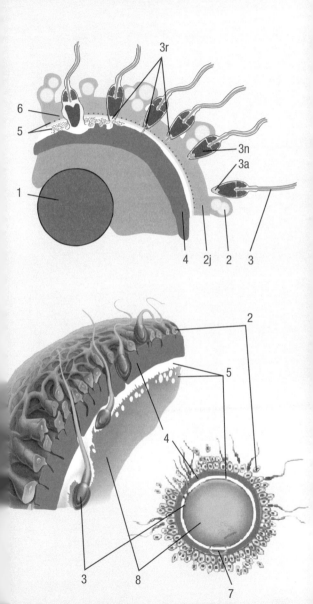

Ovary

Overview

The human ovaries are a bean shaped organs 2 X 3 X 4cm lying alongside the walls of the uterus attached to the body wall in the peritoneal cavity. They are not attached to the uterus but closely associated with it. They are whitish organs, covered with a germinal epithelium. With age, more & more follicles develop into CL, atretic follicles & corpus albicans.

1 germinal epithelium
2 stroma
3 CL wall outer theca lutein cells / inner granulosa lutein cells
4 antrum of the follicle
      a = loose CT conversion of the antrum in the CL
5 primordial follicle - in the cortex
6 medulla with BVs
7 atretic follicle
      e = early atresia
      l = late atresia
      m = moderate atresia
8 pyknotic lutein cells
9 BVs growing in from the stroma
10 CL
      e = edge of
      r = regressing
11 oöcyte + ZP
12 cumulus oophorus
13 granulosa cells
14 theca interna
15 capsule
16 corpus albicans
17 primary follicle

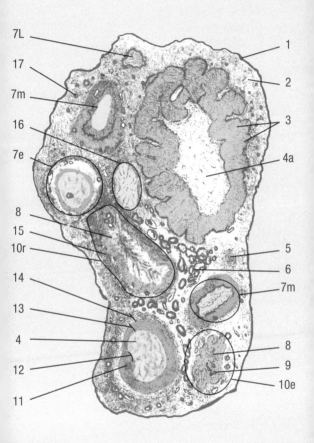

7L

17

7m

16

7e

8

15

10r

14

13

4

12

11

1

2

3

4a

5

6

7m

8

9

10e

© A. L. Neill

Ovary
Changes with Age

Microscopic views - cross-section

A   infant cortex HP

B   aging cortex MP

The infant ovary has the total amount of oöcytes a woman will ever have all as primordial follicles, approximately 1,000,000 / ovary, densely packed into the ovary cortex. By 7yo these may be reduced by half or 2/3. Further regression in the numbers occurs at puberty & with each menstral cycle when several oöcytes may begin to develop under hormonal influence, only 1 or 2 normally will do so and ovulate the others will involute regressing to form small atresic follicles, which with time begin to become a larger proportion in the ovary than the immature follicles.

By the time of the menopause most of the oöcytes will be used, but it is still possible in many women to conceive in the perimenapusal and early menopause period. Indeed this is the time when a large proportion of unplanned pregnancies do occur, due to carelessness.

The aging ovary has few immature follicles, many atresic ones & many fibrotic remains of old scarred follicles.

1   germinal epithelium

2   epithelial cord - invaginating to surround the ovum

3   developing BM - derived from the epithelial cells of the germinal epithelium, surrounding the primordial ovum (3°)

4   follicle
    e = early atretic
    L = late atretic
    p = primary

5   stroma CT

6   cortex

7   tunica albuginea - CT layer under the germinal epithelium

8   corpus albicans (fibrous replacement of the structure after the CL has regressed)

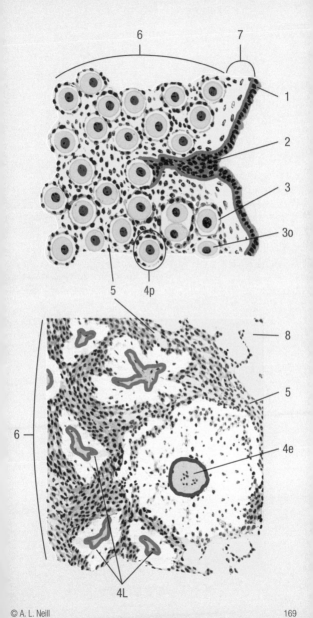

Ovary
Cell types

A follicular AKA granulosa cells
B thecal cells
C lutein cells
Schema HP

The ovary has several specialized cell types. The cells which surround the primordial follicles are the granulosa or follicular cells, derived from the germinal epithelium. They secrete mucopolysaccharides & enzymes to facilitate fluid flowing into the follicular antrum. Secondary follicles grow larger & develop multiple layers of cells compressing the stromal cells into 2 layers the theca interna cells which are vascularized & produce oestrogen & the theca externa cells. both cell types are epithelial derived although the thecal cells have many similarities to CT cells in their shape & internal structures. After ovulation the cells then form lutein cells of the CL. These cells secrete progesterone, the steroid precursor being supported in the many intracellular membranous stacks of smooth ER & vesicles. They also have multiple GA.

1 mitochondria
2 GA
3 lipid droplets
4 nucleus
    m = nuclear membrane
5 lysozymes
6 ER
    S = smooth ER
    R = rough ER (ribosomes attached)
7 nucleolus
8 vesicles

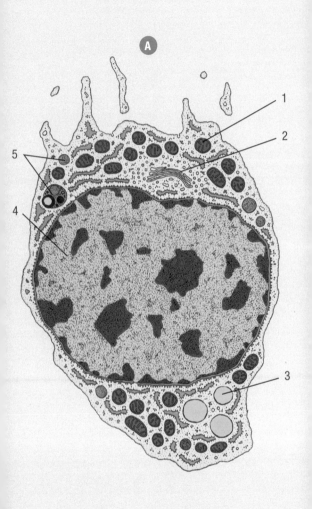

A

1

2

5

4

3

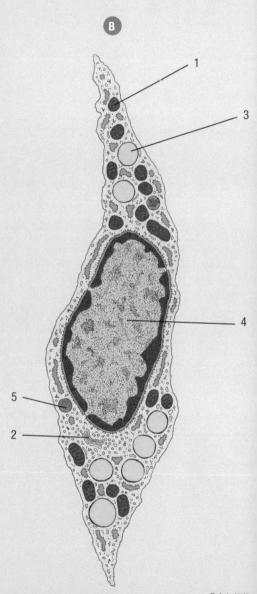

© A. L. Neill

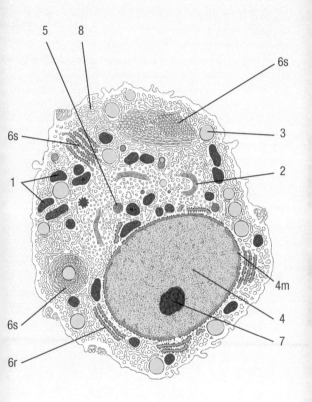

C

5 8

6s

6s

1

2

3

4m

4

7

6s

6r

Ovary
Follicle development

Macroscopic view - cross-section

The average ovary has approximately 1,000,000 germ cells, encased in surrounding stroma. Primordial follicles develop into primary follicles under hormonal influence. Fluid, follicular liquor, forms in the secondary follicle leaving the ovum surrounded by a ring of granulosa cells attached to its thickened BM AKA zona pellucida. The germinal epithelium is ruptured in ovulation. Follicles which have partially matured but do not ovulate become atretic follicles, whereas the follicle remaining after ovulation becomes the corpus luteum (CL) to support the oöcyte until fertilization occurs. It too degenerates into a small white scarred body if the oöcyte is not fertilized, the corpus albicans.

1　germinal epithelium
2　primordial follicle - in the cortex
3　epithelial cord (derived from the germinal epithelium)
4　primary follicle
5　secondary follicle
6　maturing follicle
　　　　m = mature follicle - filled with follicular liquor
7　corpus haemorrhagium AKA ruptured follicle AKA bloody body
8　CL AKA yellow body
　　　　e = early
　　　　L = late
9　medulla
10　corpus albicans AKA white body
11　ovarian BVs
12　mesovarium - CT stalk of the ovary

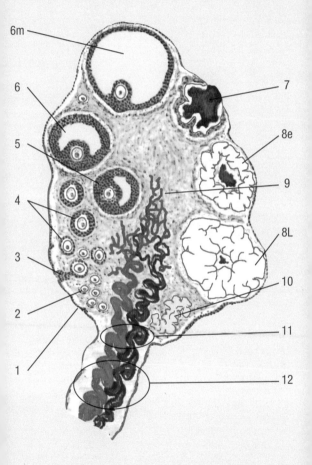

Ovary
Follicle Development

Schema from maturation to ovulation
1 primordial follicle
2 primary follicles inner & outer zones
3 secondary follicle
4 Graafian / mature follicle
5 Ovulation

Primordial follicles are arrested in prophase of the 1st meiotic division, supported by a single flattened layer of squamous follicular cells, derived from the germinal epithelium. These cells are separated from the CT stroma of the ovary by their BM. The oöcyte has several unique characteristic organelles, which include circular mitochondria & the BvB.

Primary follicles develop the ZP which interacts with the distinct cuboidal supporting follicular cells, via their microvilli. These cells differentiate into multilayered granulosa cells - strata granulosa.

Secondary follicles develop a fluid filled antrum from the rapidly growing granulosa cells & the newly formed Call-Exner bodies, expanding the follicular size & compressing the surrounding stroma into the adjacent theca interna which is vascular and produces steroids & the theca externa.

Mature Graafian follicles expand rapidly & increase in P via the growing antrum, isolating the ovum and its supporting cells from the follicular wall, so it may be expelled in ovulation.

1 stroma
2 stromal CT cells
3 BM
4 follicular cells
   s = squamous
   c = cuboidal
5 CM
6 ovum cytoplasm
7 BvB
8 lamina plates
9 ZP
10 granulosa cells - from follicular cells
11 strata granulosa
12 antrum filled with follicular liquor
13 e = theca externa
   i = theca interna
14 Call-Exner body
15 capillaries
16 cumulus orphorus - becomes the corona radiata once it leaves the follicle
17 germinal epithelium → ruptured in ovulation
18 ovum

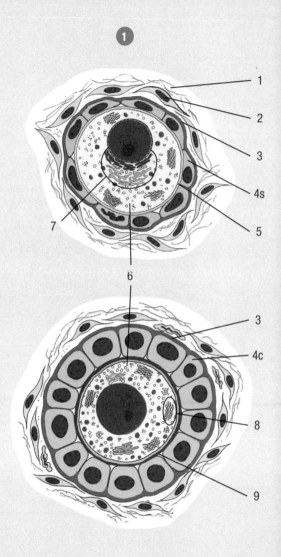

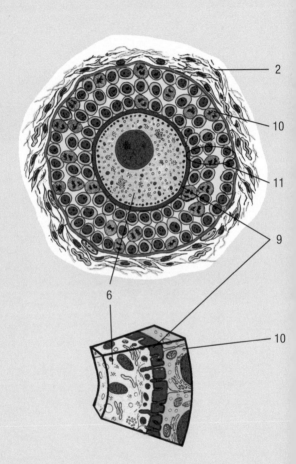

© A. L. Neil

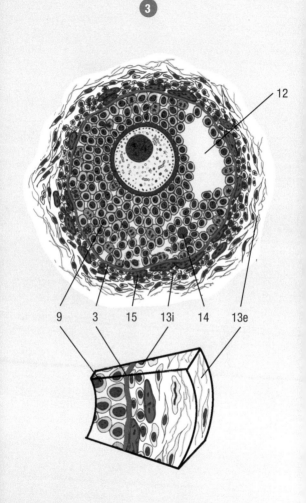

12

9   3   15   13i   14   13e

© A. L. Neill

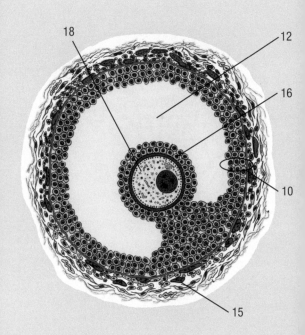

18

12

16

10

15

© A. L. Neill

18

16

17

10

12

1

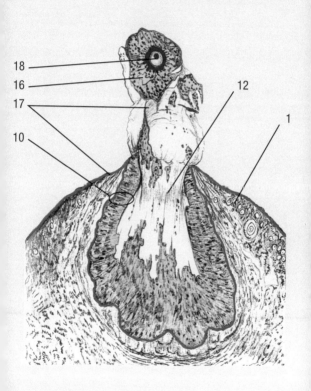

Ovarian tubes AKA Fallopian tubes
AKA Uterine tubes AKA Salpinx AKA Oviduct

Macroscopic view open (O) and closed (C) tube
Cross-sections throughout the tube

The ovarian tubes transport the ovum from the ovary to the uterus nourishing them via the goblet cells which line the walls. These tubes also facilitate the sperm entering the uterus. The egg is captured via the fimbriae as the tubes are not actually connected to the ovary. There are 3 main segments to the tube the expanded opening of the ampulla; narrows to form the isthmus, the main length of the tube to become the short contracted intramural section in the wall of the uterus.

1 ovarian tube
    a = ampulla
    i = isthmus
    w = intramural section
2 uterus
3 broad ligament
4 appendix vesiculosa
5 fimbriae

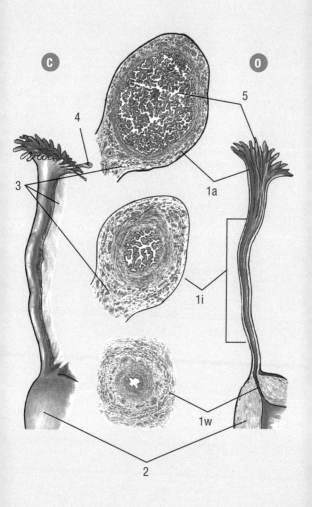

C

O

5

4

3

1a

1i

1w

2

© A. L. Neill

Ovarian tubes
Cell types

ciliated cell (A) secretory cell (B)
Schema HP

The oviducts sweep the oöcyte from the ovary to the uterus via the ciliated cells which are concentrated at the distal end of the oviduct. The environment & possibly the nutrition of the ovum are maintained by the secretory cells which are concentrated at the proximal end. They dispense their contents into the duct & then "peg out" becoming **peg cells** which protrude into the lumen (not shown here).

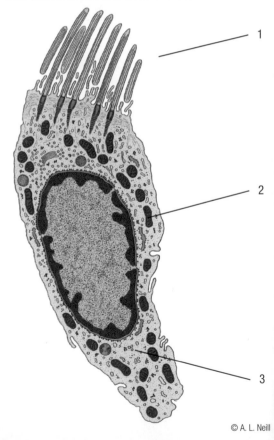

1

2

3

© A. L. Neill

1 cilia
2 nucleus
3 lysozyme
4 nucleolus
5 secretary granules mainly mucopolysaccharides
6 mv

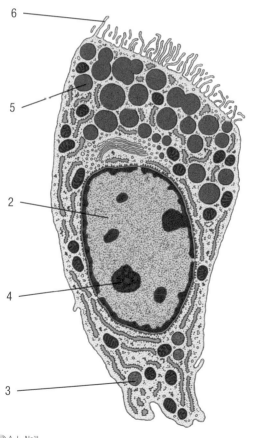

Pelvis
Bones, Joints & Internal Ligaments

A   Schema - Superior view - female
B   Macroscopic - Anterior view

The pelvis is a strong bony ring which holds the contents in via a series of strong ligaments & a muscular diaphragm. The integrity of the ligaments is essential for the maintenance of the functioning of the contained organs.

1   sacral prominence
2   rectum
3   Ileum - pelvic brim
4   ASIS
5   cervix
6   bladder
7   rectouterine lig
8   cervical lig AKA cardinal lig
9   lateral vesicular lig
10 puboivesical lig
11 superior vesicular a
12 inferior vesicular a
13 uterine a
14 inferior rectal a
15 Sacrum
16 sacral foramen
17 intervertebral disc L5/S1
18 iliosacral jt
19 Femoro-acetabular jt (hip jt)
20 PS
21 ala of the Ileum
22 ala of the SAcrum

for more details see the A to Z of Bones, Joints Ligaments & the Back

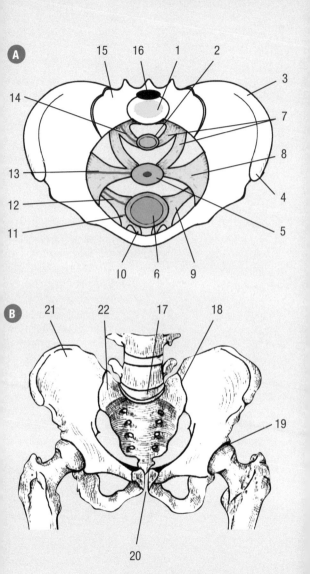

A

B

Pelvic
Contents - female

Macroscopic Anterior frontal view

1 uterus - fundus - lifted up
2 round lig
3 ovarian lig
4 ovary - lifted up from the posterior
5 infundibulopelvic lig AKA suspensory lig
6 Ileum
7 cut edge of the peritoneum
8 uterine a & v
9 cardinal lig - transporting the uterine & vaginal BVs
10 ischiorectal fossa filled with fat semi-liquid in life
11 ischiopubic ramus
12 crus of the clitoris
13 ischiocavernous m & fascia enclosing the clitoral crus c
14 superficial peroneal compartment
15 Colle's fascia
16 clitoral a
17 labia majora
18 hymen site - remnants may remain
19 posterior vaginal wall
20 vestibule of the vulva
21 labial minora
22 round lig - with fascial sheaths terminating in the Labia Majora
23 bulbourethral glands AKA Cowper's glands
24 bulbocarvernosus m + surrounding fascia
25 urogenital diaphragm containing the deep perineal muscles & their BVs
26 internal obturator m + outer obturator mem. + internal obturator fascia
27 levator ani m + its superior & inf fascia
28 ureter
29 tendinous sling
30 iliac BVs
31 infundibulum (distal end of the ovarian tube)
32 ovarian tube
33 broad lig
34 uterovaginal fascia AKA endopelvic fascia
35 cervix (AKA uterine cervix)

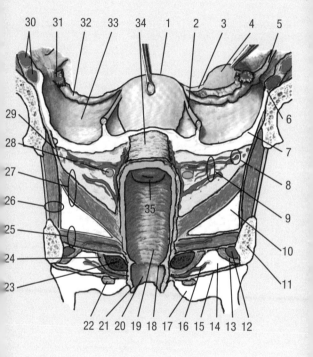

© A. L. Neill

Pelvic
Contents - female

Macroscopic

Superior view - *looking down on the pelvis*
antero- posteriorly (AP)
transverse section L 4-5

1 ureter
2 ascending colon
3 abdominal muscles - EO, IO, transversus abdominis
4 peritoneum (cut edge)
5 iliac BVs
6 suspensory lig
7 ovarian lig + ovary
8 urinary bladder + urachus - note the line of the peritoneal fold (peritoneum covers the body & posterior surface only)
9 linea alba + rectus abdominis m
10 epigastric folds of the peritoneum
11 labial BVs + round lig
12 vesicouterine pouch
13 fallopian tubes + uterus - broad lig removed
14 rectouterine pouch AKA pouch of Douglas
15 sigmoid colon
16 sacrouterine lig

Superior view - *transverse section S 1-2*

1 pelvic brim
2 obturator fascia
3 superior fascia of the pelvic diaphragm
4 uterine BVs + investing fascia
5 rectal fascia
6 common iliac BVs
7 ureter
8 sacral prominence
9 sigmoid colon
10 sacrouterine lig
11 cervix
12 obturator a + foramen
13 vesicular fascia
14 bladder - muscular fibres of the bladder AKA Detrusor m
15 urachus

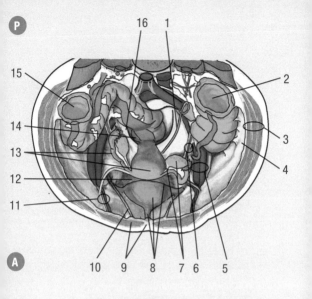

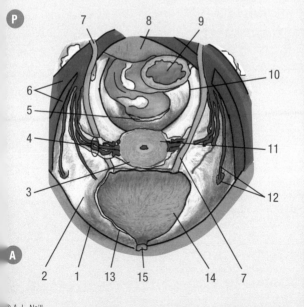

Pelvic contents - male

Macroscopic

Superior view - *looking down on the pelvis*
antero- posteriorly (AP)
transverse section L 4-5

1 ureter
2 ascending colon
3 abdominal muscles
    e = EO,
    i = IO,
    t = transversus abdominus
4 peritoneum (cut edge)
5 iliac BVs
6 urinary bladder + urachus - note the line of the peritoneal fold (peritoneum covers the body & posterior surface only)
7 linea alba + rectus abdominis m
8 epigastric folds of the peritoneum
9 rectovesical pouch
10 sigmoid colon

P

1
2
3e
3
4
3i
5
3t

10
9

8   7   6

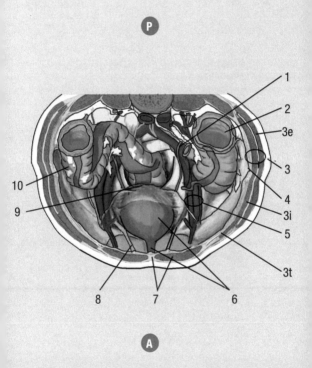

A

© A. L. Neill

Pelvis
Pelvic diaphragm - female

Musculature
Macroscopic A *Inferior view*
              B *Internal view of the lateral wall*
              C *External view of the medial wall -*
                 Ileum cut away
              D *Superior view*

The inferior border of the pelvis is the pelvic diaphragm - a basin of skeletal muscle which supports the pelvic contents. The 3 passages which pass through the female pelvis are intimately connected via interdigitating muscle & CT fibres. These allow for the change in shape necessary to pass substances, while still maintaining continence. Any displacement or forward movement of the superior structures may upset this fine P balance and affect the passage of all substances.

1 PS	13 piriformis m
2 urethral opening + musculofascical extension	14 Sacrum f = foramen
3 vaginal opening + musculofascical extension	15 Coccyx
	16 coccygeus m

4   levator ani m
     a = pubococcygeus m
     b = iliiococcygeus m
	17 dorsal v of the clitoris

	18 suprapubic lig
	19 pelvic brim
5 ischiopubic ramus	20 obturator foramen / canal
6 interdigitating fibres of the perineal body	21 transverse pelvic lig
7 rectum + musculofascical extension covered by the EAS	22 urogenital diaphragm - inf + sup. fascial layers enclosing muscle
8 tendinous arch	23 supf. peroneal m
9 obturator internus m	24 EAS covers the musculofascial extension

10   Ischium
     s = ischeal spine
     t = ischeal tuberosity
	25 Colle's fascia

	26 Pubis
	27 dorsal vein of the clitoris
11 sacrotuberous lig c = cut edges	28 sacrococcygeal lig
	29 sacral lig + iliosacral lig
12 sacrospinous lig c = cut edges	30 sacral promintary
	31 inguinal lig
	32 subpubic lig

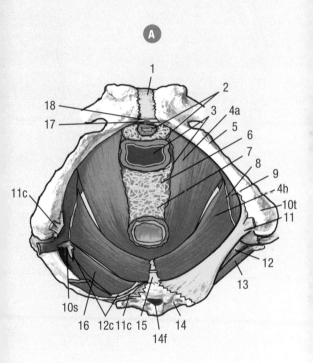

A

1

18
17

2
3 4a
5
6
7
8
9
4b
10t
11

11c

12
13

10s
16 12c 11c 15   14
          14f

© A. L. Neill

195

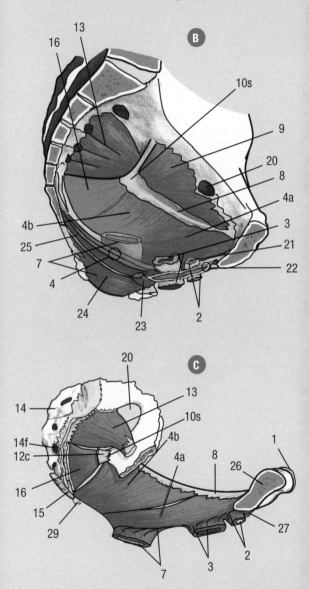

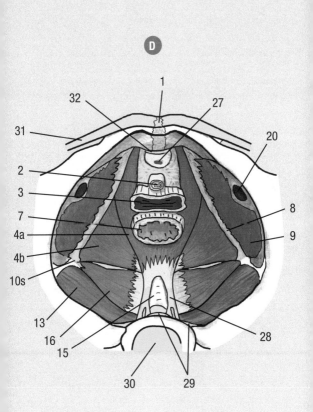

Pelvic Examination

A Uterus examination

With an empty bladder (void before the examination) the vaginal fingers push the cervix back & up fixing it (f) so it is possible to examine the fundus (e) through the abdomen. Fixing (f) the fundus after examination - the ant. surface of the cervix may be (e) in the vagina.

B Adnexal mass examination (ovarian)

Placing a hand in the vaginal fornix of each side push laterally & with the abdominal hand palpate for an adnexial mass on each side - only enlarged masses can be detected this way.

C Examination of enterocele / rectocele

Entering from the rectum the finger is able to track through the sac protruding into the vagina in the rectocele. This is not possible in the enterocele.

1 vagina
2 small intestine
3 uterus
4 rectum

D Examination of the perineum and integrity of the perineal body

To assess the integrity of the perineal body and structures of the perineum, place fingers in the rectum & vagina palpate the T in b/n.

5 perineal body

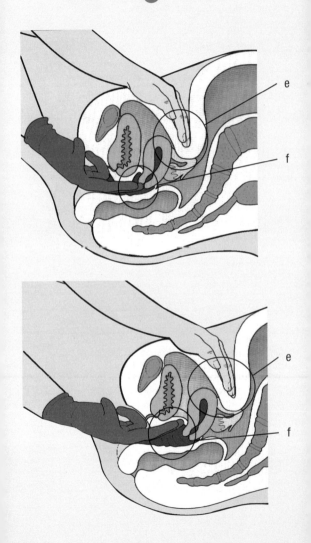

e

f

e

f

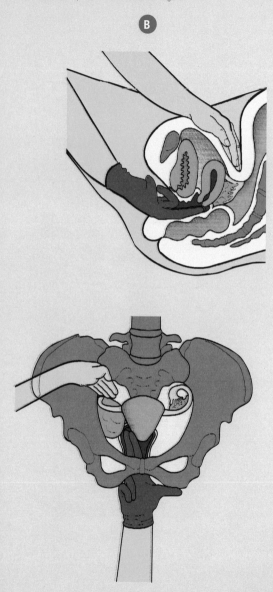

© A. L. Neill

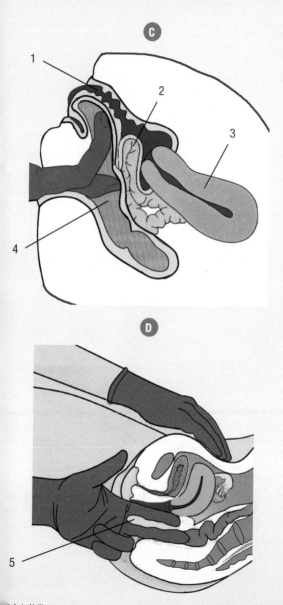

Penis
Shaft

Histology - Transverse section
A   LP H&E overview of the penile shaft
B   HP H&E penile urethra

The shaft of the penis has 2 major functions: to carry the urine and the ejaculate. It consists of 3 "spongy" bodies covered with several layers of CT, which have the capacity to become engorged with arterial blood, expand, enlarge and harden. This supports the passage of the ejaculate so that it is able to be placed as close as possible to the site of fertilization.

1   dorsal penile v
     d = deep
     s = superficial
2   dorsal penile a & N
3   deep a
4   cavernous sinus of corpus cavernosa
5   helicine a
6   tunica albuginea cavernosa containing CT & M
7   urethra in the corpus spongiosum
8   tunica albuginea spongiosa
9   cavernous sinus of corpus spongiosum
10 lining transitional epithelium
11 deep penile fascia with BVs (Buck's fascia)
12 dermis and epidermis
13 Dartos tunic - thin CT covered muscle
14 corpus cavernosa
15 urethral gland of Littre + duct
16 trabeculae (supporting the sinuses)
17 lamina propria
18 BVs of the corpus spongiosum
19 sebaceous glands

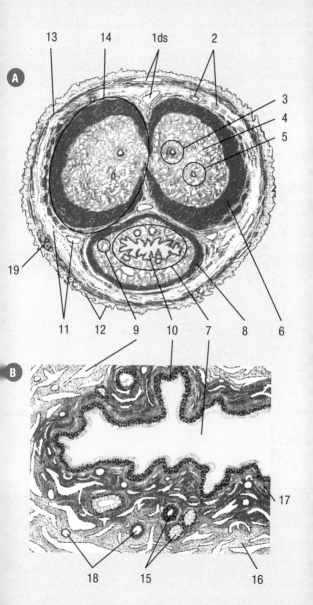

Penis

Macroscopic view
A showing the 3 main components
B sagittal section showing the floor of the penis

1 glans penis
2 corpus cavernosum
3 pubic bone
4 ischeal tuberosity
5 deep transverse perinei m
6 central lig
7 corpus spongiosum
8 bulbourethral glands
9 deep artery of the penis
10 penile urethra
11 opening of the bulbourethral glands

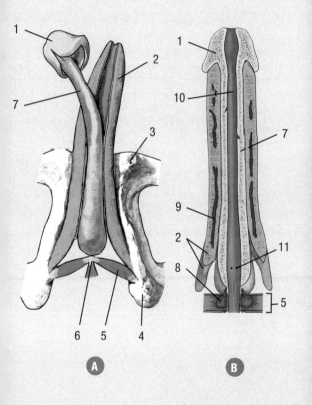

Perineum
Triangles - female & male

Macroscopic   Inferior views
*   Female*
*   Male - genitalia moved anteriorly*
Schema - inferior & sagittal views

The perineum is divided into 2 angled triangles which have their
centre through the PB. The urogenital triangle supports the external
genitalia (U) - vulva in the female - & the anal triangle (A) supports
the levator ani muscle group & the anus. The anterior border is the
PS; the posterior the Coccyx & laterally it is bounded by the Ischeal
Tuberosities. The lowest point is the PB which forms the base of both
triangles.

A = anal triangle
U = urogenital triangle

1   pubic arch
2   Coccyx
3   sacrotuberous lig
4   ischeal tuberosity
5   perineal body (PB)
6   anus
7   Pubis

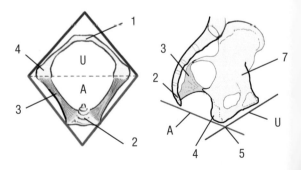

© A. L. Ne

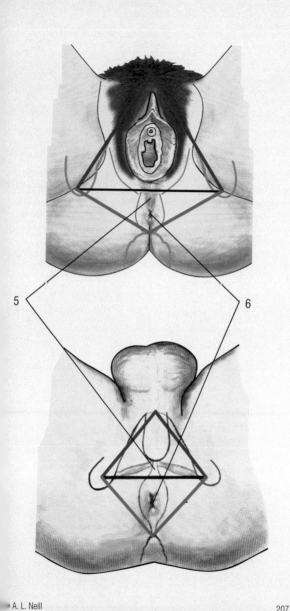

5

6

A. L. Neill

Perineum
Blood Supply - Female

Macroscopic   Inferior view
deep dissection superficial structures removed

The perineum is defined as the surface region in both males and females b/n the pubic symphysis & the coccyx. It is bounded by the pelvic diaphragm superiorly, the legs laterally and the skin inferiorly. It is a diamond-shaped area on the inferior surface of the trunk that includes all the passages exiting the body, through the pelvic outlet, which are intimately related, often sharing common walls . Hence injury to one may impact on the control of the other passages, with severe consequences.

1   dorsal a of the clitoris
2   crus of the clitoris
3   deep artery of the clitoris
4   vestibular bulb + Bartholin's gland
5   clitoral a
6   internal pudendal a
7   sacrotuberous lig
8   inferior haemorrhoidal a
9   anus + EAS
10 anococcygeal body
11 coccyx
12 PB - central lig
13 gluteus maximus m
14 ischiorectal fossa
15 ischeal tuberosity
16 supf. transverse peroneal m + perineal a
17 supf. peroneal fascia - the most inferior but closest to the skin
18 pubic ramus b
19 ischiocavernosis m
20 vagina
21 mons pubis
22 external urethral orifice

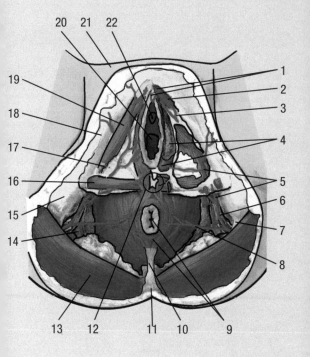

Urogenital diaphragm
Male

Macroscopic Inferior view
> *A Looking into the Deep pouch*
> *B Looking onto the Superficial pouch*

The urogenital diaphragm is the fascial supportive layer of the urogenital triangle and it permits the passage of the urethra in the male. Sandwiched b/n 2 strong fascial layers are glands and muscles which contribute to the ejaculate.

1 PS
2 Pubis b
3 superior pubic ramus
4 deep dorsal vein of the penis
5 inf. fascia of the urogenital diaphragm
6 dorsal a & N of the penis
7 ischeal tuberosity
8 cut surface of Colle's fascia
9 transverse peroneal m
>   d = deep
>   s = superficial
10 urethra + sphincter (s)*
11 Bulbourethral glands + ducts AKA Cowper's glands
12 ischiopubic ramus b
13 transverse pelvic lig
14 arcuate lig of the pubis
15 deep artery of the penis
16 urethral a
17 central body of the perineum
18 fusion of the deep & supf fascia of the urogenital diaphragm

* note the thickness much stronger than the female equivalent & a complete circle unlike in the female. It also encompasses the duct of the Cowper's glands

© A. L. Ne

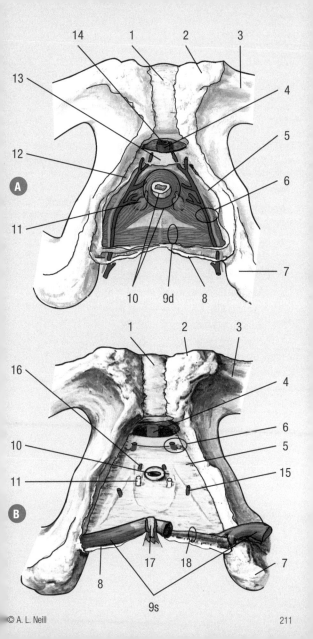

Urogenital triangle
Female

Macroscopic Inferior view

      A Superficial pouch

      B Deep pouch

The urogenital triangle is one of the 2 triangles of the perineum - it supports the external genitalia in the female this includes: the clitoris, urethra & vagina, which pass through the strong fascial support diaphragm.

1 PS
2 urethra
3 deep peroneal cavity
4 urethral sphincter m
5 inf. fascia of the urogenital diaphragm
6 deep transverse peroneal m
7 vaginal cavity
8 Bartholin's gland
9 ischiopubic ramus b
10 vestibular bulb
11 crus of the clitoris
12 clitoris shaft & glans

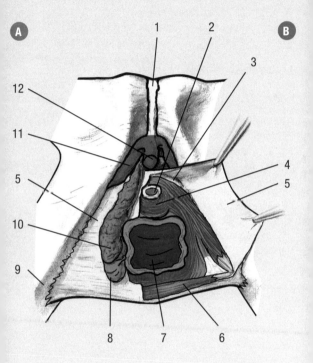

A

B

Perineum
Musculature - Female

Macroscopic - inferior view

The pelvic contents are supported anteriorly by the pelvic diaphragm: a strong CT sheet with embedded muscles permitting the passage of the urethra and the vagina. Posteriorly the contents are supported by the levator ani; a movable muscular wall supporting the sigmoid colon & rectum. This is by far the more flexible and allows for the passage of varying volumes of material w/o compromising the structure or support basis.

1 clitoris
2 urethral & vaginal openings
3 inf. pubic ramus
4 ischiocavernosis m
5 bulbospongiosis m
6 perineal membrane part of the urogenital diaphragm
7 supf. transverse peroneal m
8 sacrotuberous lig
9 levator ani m - composed of
    a = pubococcygeus m
    b = puborectalis m
    c = iliococcygeal m
10 gluteus maximus m
11 Colles' fascia
12 EAM
    a = subcutaneous
    b = superficial
    c = deep
13 obturator internus m
14 deep peroneal fascia AKA Gallauder's fascia
15 PB

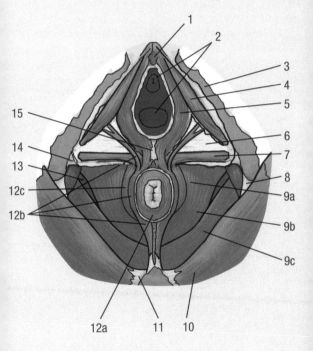

Perineum
Musculature - Male

Macroscopic - inferior view

The pelvic contents are supported anteriorly by the pelvic diaphragm: a strong CT sheet with embedded muscles permitting the passage of the urethra. Posteriorly the contents are supported by the levator ani; a movable muscular wall supporting the sigmoid colon & rectum. This is by far the more flexible and allows for the passage of varying volumes of material w/o compromising the structure or support basis.

1 shaft of the penis
2 midline raphe
3 inf. pubic ramus
4 ischiocavernosis m
5 bulbospongiosis m
6 perineal membrane
7 supf. transverse peroneal m
8 sacrotuberous lig
9 levator ani m - composed of
    a = pubococcygeus m
    b = puborectalis m
    c = iliococcygeal m
10 gluteus maximus m
11 Colles' fascia
12 EAS
    a = subcutaneous
    b = superficial
    c = deep
13 obturator internus m
14 deep peroneal fascia AKA Gallauder's fascia
15 PB

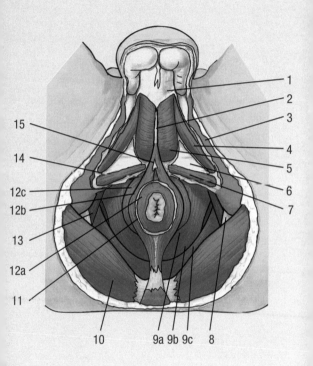

15

14

12c

12b

13

12a

11

1

2

3

4

5

6

7

10   9a 9b 9c   8

Pineal gland AKA Epiphysis Cerebri AKA The Third eye

Macroscopic view
Sagittal section through part of the brain

The pineal gland is a pine cone shaped gland of diencephalon (6X6mm). It has a strong BS considering its small size, and acts as a bridge b/n the nervous & endocrine systems similar to the Hypothalamus / Pituitary glands, converting sensory input of the SymNS to H signals.   The main H produced is Melatonin. The pineal gland influences: sexual development, the onset of menarche & menopause, male puberty & the body's circadian rhythm (sleep wake cycle). It is photosensitive, despite being in the centre of the brain. It often calcifies with age, & accumulates fluoride selectively. The effect on its function in these circumstances is not known.

1 corpus callosum
2 choroid plexus of 3rd ventricle
3 intermediate mass of the thalamus
4 commissure
    a = anterior
    p = posterior
5 optic chiasm
6 hypothalamus
7 pituitary gland
8 mammillary body
9 pons
10 cerebral aqueduct
11 cerebellum
12 superior cervical sympathetic ganglia
13 sympathetic input to the pineal gland
14 pineal gland

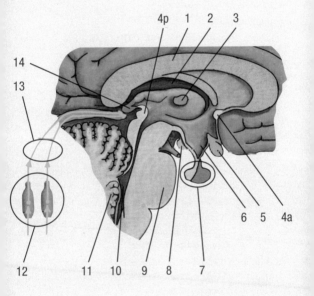

Pituitary gland

Schema overview

1. hypothalamus - neurons interact with the cells &/or BVs of the pituitary gld directly to affect its secretions
2. primary capillary plexus
3. optic chiasm
4. pituitary portal system
5. pituitary gland
   - a = ant. pituitary AKA adenohypophysis
   - p = post. pituitary AKA neurohypophysis
6. basophilic cells secrete
   - a = ACTH - stimulates the adrenal gld
   - b = TSH - stimulates the thyroid
   - c = FSH - stimulates maturation of ovary follicles & oestrogen secretion
   - c = FSH - stimulates spermatogenesis
   - d = LH - stimulates ovulation
   - d = LH - stimulates testosterone secretion
7. acidophilic cells secrete
   - a = prolactin - stimulates milk secretion
   - b = GH - causes hyperglycaemia
     - elevates free fatty acids
     - stimulates bone growth
8. neurohypophyseal cells secrete
   - a = oxytocin - causes uterine contractions & milk ejection
   - b = ADH - causes water retention

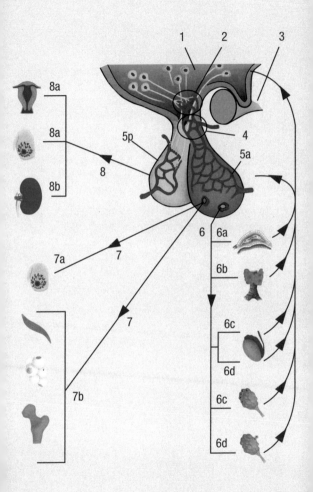

Prostate gland & Prostatic urethra

Histology

MP H&E showing relationship b/n the urethra and the prostate gland

The prostate organ is a lobular exocrine gland divided by fibromuscular septa. The 3 main lobes surround the male urethra, emptying their contents into it along with the ejaculate. Most of the sperm are suspended in the secretion which nourishes and supports them along with the secretions of the seminal vesicles. The sub-urethral glands of the posterior lobe often undergo hypertrophy with age compressing the trigone area of the bladder and restrict emptying.

1   utricle (male equivalent of the uterus) post. to the urethra
2   prostatic ducts
3   fibromuscular stroma surrounding the gland
4   concretions w/in the prostatic glands
5   prostate glands
6   smooth m in the stroma
7   ejaculatory ducts
8   prostatic sinuses
9   prostatic urethra - lined with transitional epithelium

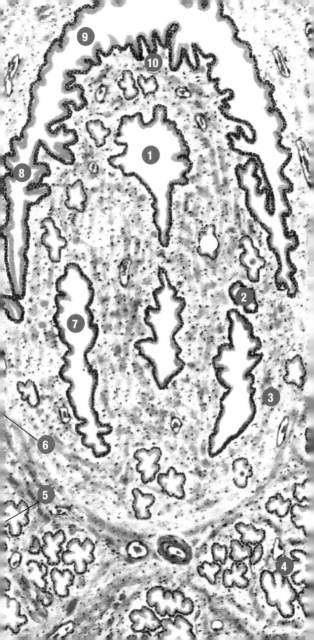

Prostate gland

Histology
HP H&E showing the internal glandular structure

The prostate organ is a lobular exocrine gland divided by fibromuscular septa. The 3 main lobes surround the male urethra, emptying their contents into it along with the ejaculate. Most of the sperm are suspended in the secretion which nourishes and supports them along with the secretions of the seminal vesicles. The sub-urethral glands of the posterior lobe often undergo hypertrophy with age compressing the trigone area of the bladder and restrict emptying.

1 excretory ducts
2 smooth muscle bands
3 acini of the prostatic glands
4 columnar epithelium lining the glands
5 concretions w/in the prostatic glands
6 prostatic secretions
7 CT fibrous folds
8 BVs

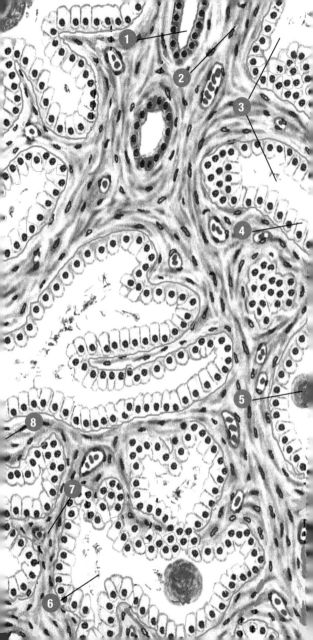

Prostate gland

Macroscopic view

A   Coronal section anterior tissue removed

*B   Transverse section showing the relationship b/n the
urethra and the prostate gland*

The prostate gland is a lobular exocrine gland responsible for the
nutrition of the sperm in the ejaculate. Its secretions help to neutralize
the acid vaginal environment and prolong the life of the sperm. It wraps
itself around the urethra and sits on the muscles of the pelvic floor.

1   bladder internal surface - note cords of smooth m
     hypertrophy due to difficulty in emptying from protrusion
     by the posterior lobe

2   lateral lobe of the prostate gland

3   prostatic urethra

4   opening for the utricle (midline)

5   posterior prostatic lobe protruding into the bladder
     trigone area
         note sub-urethral ducts

6   anterior lobe

7   capsule - actually the fibromuscular coat which separates
     and surrounds each lobe

8   ejaculatory glands

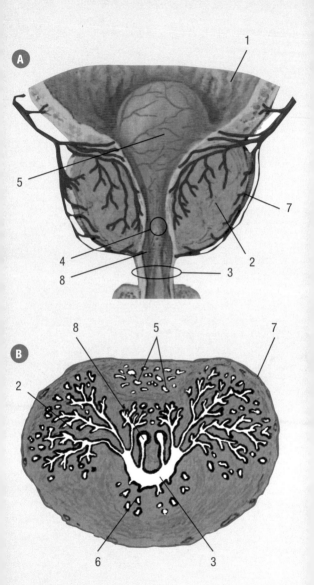

Prostate gland

Schema
comparing zonal with lobar anatomy
cross section of the gland showing the zones
outline of the ducts of the gland and their relationship with the urethra

The prostate organ can be divided into lobes macroscopically, or zones functionally. The hormonal influence of the glands growth/hypertrophy is zonal rather than lobular, as is the gland type.

1 urethra
2 ejaculatory ducts
3 utricle (male equivalent of the utuerus) post. to the urethra

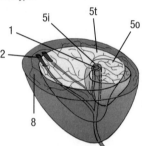

4 prostatic ducts of the
      a = anterior lobe
      L = lateral lobe
      m = median lobe
      p = posterior lobe
      s = suburethral region (part of the posterior lobe)

5 periurethral zone - glands here enter the urethra directly and are predominantly mucosal
      i = inner or suburethral
      o = outer
      t = transitional - ill defined area b/n the 2

6 fibromuscular capsule - the smooth m contents are significant in emptying the gland when stimulated
7 CT septa and supporting stroma
8 peripheral zone - glands here enter the urethra via long ducts

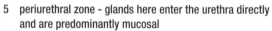

© A. L. Neill

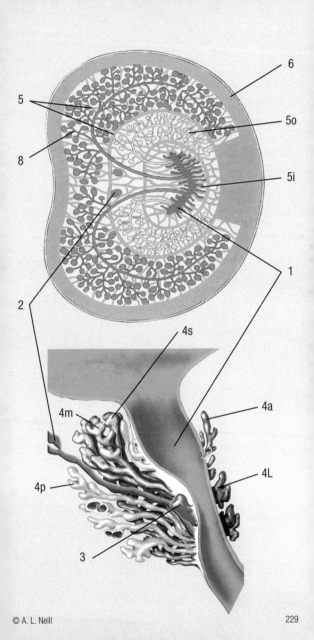

Pudendal Nerve

Schema - Male

A   superiolateral view

B   inferior view

The Pudendal N (S2,3,4) is a mixed N with branches which supplies the penis & scrotum in the male and vulva in the female. Its major branches are : the inferior rectal AKA inferior haemorrhoidal N, post. scrotal (labial) N; dorsal N to the [penis (clitoris). It also supplies: levator ani m, EAS, coccygeus m & muscles of the ant. perineum, as well as the skin covering these areas.

1 perineal br
2 posterior scrotal (labial) Ns
3 dorsal N to the penis (clitoris)
4 EAS + levator ani m & its N
5 supf. post. scrotal (labial) Ns
6 deep post. scrotal (labial) Ns
7 transversus perineal superficialis m
8 N to bulbospongiosus m
9 N to ischiocavernosus m
10 N to transverse perineal profundus m
11 N to sphincter urethrae m
12 Spinal roots S 234
13 lumbosacral plexus
14 urethra
15 Coccyx + coccygeus m
16 ischeal tuberosity

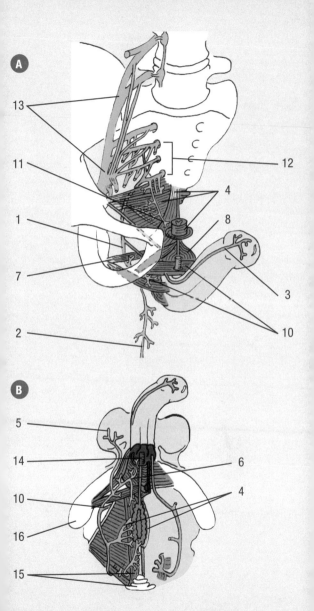

13

11

1

7

2

12

4

8

3

10

5

14

10

16

15

6

4

© A. L. Neill

Seminal vesicle

Macrosopic view

Posterio-inferior to show the relations with the bladder & prostate

The bladder and inf. structures have been forwardly displaced from the pelvic diaphragm to show the passage & position of urethra

The seminal vesicles are paired, highly coiled, tubular structures superior to the prostate, posterior to the bladder. They merge with the Vas deferens, which becomes continuous with the prostatic urethra. As with most of the urogenital system the tube is lined with transitional epithelium, with a surrounding thick fibromuscular tunica.

The prostate gland, seminal vesicles and bulbourethral glands (Cowper's glands) all have input into the seminal fluid, feeding & sustaining the sperm.

1   bladder -full, showing muscle bands, peritoneal covering has been removed
2   ureter
3   ductus deferens = vas deferens
4   ampulla of the ductus deferens
5   seminal vesicle
6   prostate gland
7   ischiopubic ramus of the pelvic girdle
8   bulbourethral glands
9   muscles of the urogenital diaphragm
10 urethra
11 fascia of the urogenital diaphragm

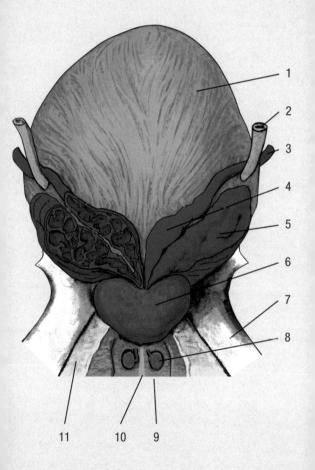

Seminiferous epithelium

Schema

HP of the cell types of spermatogenesis

The epithelium of the seminiferous tubules is the site of spermatogenesis. The more differentiated the cells the closer they become to the lumen and then when mature break off and are collected via ductules to the epididymus.

1 late spermatid
2 early spermatid
3 primary spermatocyte
4 junctional complex b/n sertoli cells
5 BM
6 sertoli cells - support cells of the developing sperm
7 peritubular myoepithelial cells
8 type A - pale spermatogonium = stem cell
9 type B - dark spermatogonium = going to become differentiated germ cells AKA sperm
10 residual bodies
11 acrosome

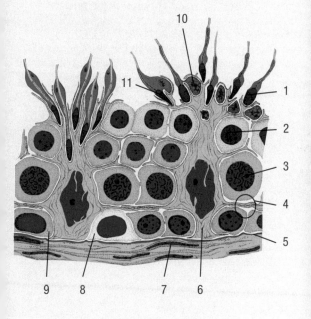

Sex act AKA Coitus AKA Intercourse AKA Vaginal sex

Schema

A LP

B HP

The definition of sex has been debated extensively, but coitus generally means penile-vaginal penetration, for the purpose of reproduction & or sexual pleasure. For fertilization to occur the penis must be in contact with the vagina; and there must also be an uninterrupted passage from the testis to the uterus & the ovarian tubes. Meanwhile the ovum must be swept into the fallopian tubes from the ovary, and move along the tubes to meet the sperm.

Note the pathway for the ejaculate and the urine to exit is the same but due to the external P on the bladder at times of intercourse, the bladder is unable to empty at that time.

1 seminal vesicle
2 vas deferens
    a = ampulla
3 clitoris
4 uterus
5 ovary
6 opening of ovarian tube
7 cervix
8 glans penis - head of the penis
9 urethra - penile segment
10 penis shaft + vaginal introitus & wall
11 testis
12 epididymis
13 urethra - pelvic segment
14 prostate gland
15 bladder

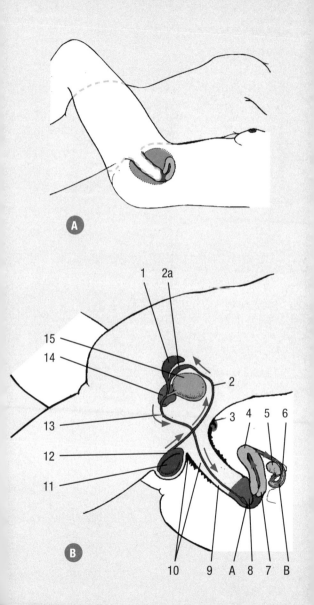

Sexual Response Cycle - Female

Schema

The sexual response cycle has 4 phases in the female.

A - THE EXCITEMENT PHASE

physical &/or psychological stimulation - for mins → hrs
sexual flush -erythematosus morbilliform skin change over the chest, neck & face
- the breasts enlarge, the nipples become erect, BP ↑ , HR ↑ , muscle tone ↑

  1a The uterus elevates
  2a The clitoris enlarges
  3a The labia swell
  4a The vagina lubricates

B - THE PLATEAU PHASE

the breasts continue to enlarge, BP ↑ , HR ↑ , muscle tone ↑

  1b The uterus elevates further, & the cervix opens slightly to allow for
      better passage of the sperm
  2b The clitoris becomes erect & the hood retreats
  3b The labia swell & become engorged
  4b The Bartholin's glands secrete fluid & the vagina enlarges

C - THE ORGASMIC PHASE

THIS MAY BE REPEATED SEVERAL TIMES BEFORE MOVING ONTO THE NEXT
PHASE

there is a release of sexual tension with a peak of BP ↑ , HR ↑ , muscle
tone ↑ but loss of voluntary muscle tone & RR ↑↑

  1c uterine & lower abdominal & anal muscles contract 1/sec > 15
  2c peak sensitivity in the clitoris & other genital erogenous zones
  3c labia are well lubricated and engorged
  4c vaginal muscle contractions synchronized with the other
      contractions

D - THE RESOLUTION PHASE

the breast & nipples return to normal, BP HR become normal & sexual flush
disappears

  1d uterus returns to normal position
  2d clitoris returns to normal
  3d labia return to normal
  4d vagina returns to normal tone & size, lubrication stops

Sexual Response Cycle - Male

Schema

The sexual response cycle has 5 phases in the male.

A - THE EXCITEMENT PHASE

physical &/or psychological stimulation - for mins ➝ hrs
the nipples & penis become erect, blood pools in the extremities BP ↑,
HR ↑, muscle tone ↑

  1a The penis becomes erect
  2a The testis swell & elevate

B - THE PLATEAU PHASE

the sexual flush appears on the chest BP ↑, HR ↑, muscle tone ↑

  1b The penis may become harder
  2b The testes swell by 50%
  3b The Cowper's glands secrete fluid - the pre-ejaculate (this may
      contain sperm)
  4b prostate enlarges

C - THE ORGASMIC PHASE

there is a release of sexual tension with a peak of BP ↑, HR ↑, muscle
tone ↑ but loss of voluntary muscle tone & RR ↑↑

  1c the penis **point of imminence** occurs - when an orgasm
      &ejaculation is inevitable -
  2c rhythmic contractions occur in the VD & seminal vesicles,
  3c urethral contractions occur the initial ones being the strongest &
      these push the semen into & through the urethra & expel it
  4c prostate gland contracts
  5c bladder is prevented from emptying due to P at its base by the
      prostate

D - THE RESOLUTION PHASE

the BP HR & RR return to normal & sexual flush disappears

  1d penis deflates
  2d testes descend

E - REFRACTORY PERIOD

Not shown this phase prevents back to back orgasms as there must be a
recovery and restoration of the penile function lasts min ➝ hrs <30yo, hrs ➝
days >50yo; increasing with age & decreasing levels of testosterone

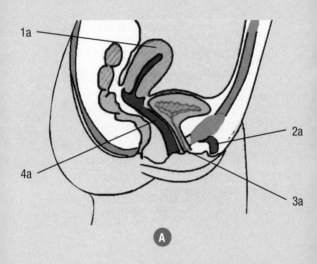

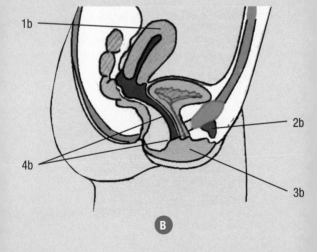

© A. L. Neil

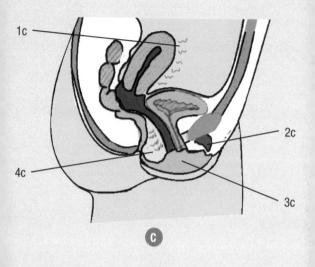

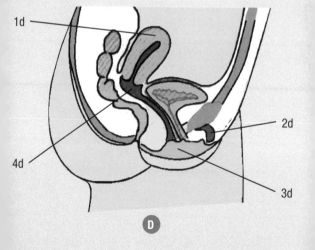

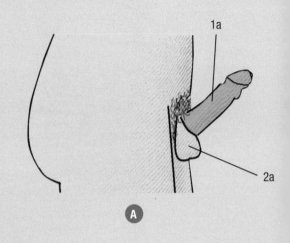

1a

2a

A

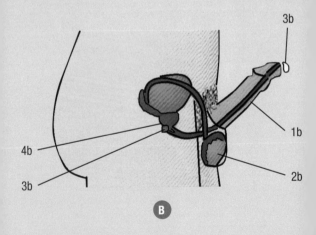

3b

1b

4b

3b

2b

B

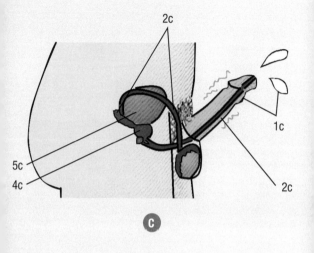

C

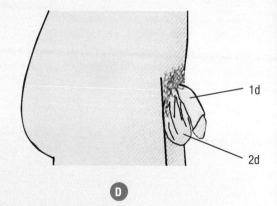

D

Spermatogenesis

Schema

A   Stem cells - type A spermatogonia - do not differentiate

*B   Progenitor cells - type B spermatogonia - multiply &
differentiate*

C   meiotic division first & second

*D   Spermiogenesis - differentiation from spermatid to
spermatozoa*

Spermatogenesis is the process by which spermatozoa are formed
from the original male germ cell the spermatogonium. At puberty
- male sexual maturity the germ cells undergo mitosis. Some
remain as germ cells = type A spermatogonia; while others begin to
differentiate = type B spermatogonia, ultimately forming the primary
spermatocytes, which then do not divide but differentiate into the
specialized spermatozoa, when they finally cleave their cytoplasmic
connecting bridge.

1   mitosis

2   primary spermatocytes - undergo the first meiotic division

3   secondary spermatocytes undergo the second meiotic
division - now haploid

4   cells of this pathway are all connected by a cytoplasmic
bridge unit the cleavage and release of 5

5   mature spermatozoa - free floating cleavage of the
cytoplasmic bridge & ...

6   residual bodies (similar to the polar bodies of the ova)

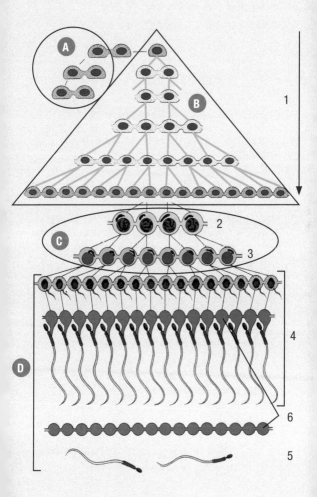

Spermatogenesis

Spermiogenesis

Schema

Di *Spermatid*

Dii *Golgi phase - prominent development of the GA*

Diii *Acrosomal phase*

Div *Maturation phase*

Once the spermatids are formed the cells no longer undergo division but differentiate into the spermatozoa. These small cells (7-8μm) are close to the lumen in the seminiferous tubules, moving closer with further development; which consists of the formation of the acrosome, condensation & elongation of the nucleus, formation of the flagellum and the shedding of most of the cytoplasm. This takes place over 3 stages.

The whole process takes b/n 70-90 days and is not regulated as in the female. This means sperm are always present & available for fertilization but that any disruption in the process of this development may take up to 3 months to regularize.

7 GA

8 acrosome

    c = cap

    g = granule

9 centrioles - forming the developing flagellum - pulls it into the nucleus

10 nucleus

    c = concentrated nuclear material

    v = vacuoles

11 cytoplasm

    c = concentrated

    r = residual cytoplasm - will form residual bodies

12 manchette (becomes post acromal sheath)

13 flagellum

14 mitochondria

    s = mitochondrial sheath

15 annular ring

16 fibrous sheath

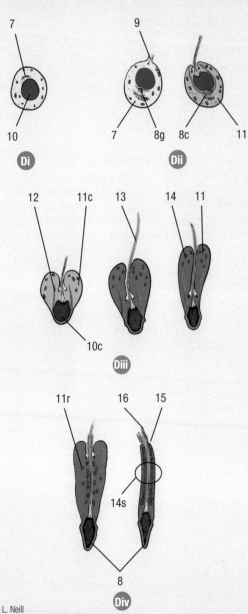

Spermatogenesis

Spermatazoa

Schema

A   Head = 5μm   *(frontal & sagittal views)*

B   *Middle piece = 5μm*

C   *Principal piece = 50μm -*

D   *End piece = 5μm*

Tail = C + D

The flagellum and large numbers of the mitochondria in the middle piece ensure that the sperm is very motile and able to traverse long distances, in order to meet the ovum. Energy is also needed to pierce the ZP of the ovum and release the nuclear contents into the cytoplasm of the egg. The unique shape of the sperm facilitates these activities.

17 neck

18 axonemal complex - consisting of
- i = inner central pair of microfilaments
- o = outer 9 doublets of dense fibres
- m = central mass

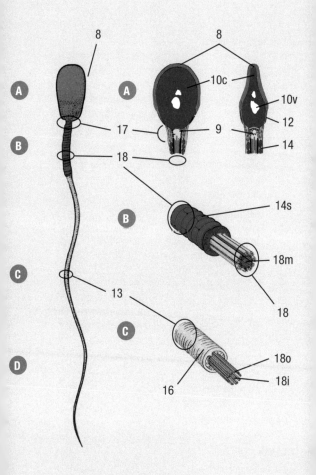

Testes and Spermatic cord

A Schema of the spermatic cord & testis
B Schema of Testis
C Inguinal ligament

The testes are the male equivalent of the ovaries. They begin in the abdominal cavity outside the peritoneum and progress down out of the body via the Gubernaculum (female equivalent round lig in the Labia Majora) through the layers of the abdomen which are reflected in the layers of the connecting spermatic cord, and end up in the scrotal sac (female equivalent Labia Majora). Descent of the testes at puberty is essential for fertility.

1   deep inguinal ring
2   superficial inguinal ring - from which the spermatic cord emerges
3   spermatic cord

	testicular layer	abdominal wall equivalent
4	Dartos m in the subcutaneous fascia (much the same as the muscles of expression)	Scarpa's fascia
5	External spermatic fascia	External abdominal oblique m
6	Cremaster m	Internal abdominal oblique m
7m		Transversus abdominus m
7	Internal spermatic fascia	Transverse fascia
8	Tunica vaginalis - parietal	Peritoneum
9	Tunica vaginalis - visceral	Peritoneum

10   testis
      d = descended
      u = undescended
11   skin + subcutaneous fascia
12   ductus deferens AKA vas deferens
13   peritoneum
14   ilioinguinal N
15   inguinal lig
16   pectineal + lacunar lig
17   obliterated umbilical folds & arteries
18   inferior epigastric art

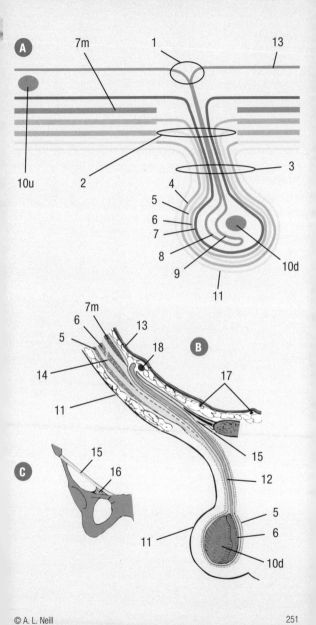

Testes

Macroscopic view
Anterior with penis elevated and anterior tissue layers removed

The testes are the male equivalent of the ovaries. They begin in the abdominal cavity and progress down out of the body connected by the spermatic cord into the scrotal sac. This is necessary because spermatogenesis will not occur at body temperature. If the testes do not descend (cryptorchidism) after puberty, they become sterile.

1   shaft of the penis
2   frenulum (note this is a circumcised penis)
3   testis covered by tunia vaginalis - visceral layer
4   epididymis
      a = appendix of epididymis
5   spermatic cord
6   ductus deferens AKA vas deferens (with the artery of the vas deferens)
7   pampiniform venous plexus
8   internal spermatic artery
9   cremaster m
10 dartos m

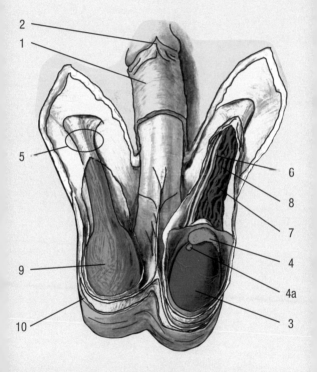

Testes

Macroscopic view
Sagittal section showing interior & BS
Schema of tubules to show continuity from the testis

The testes are the site of spermatogenesis. The sperm once matured breakaway from the epithelial lining of the seminiferous tubules from which they are derived & proceed to the epididymis, & then through to the VD to the seminal vesicles.

1 vas deferens
2 epididymis
     d = ductus epididyis
3 vasa efferentes
4 vas aberans
5 tunica albuginea
6 fibrous septum
7 lobule
8 rete testis in the mediastinum of the testis
9 pampiniform plexus
10 internal spermatic artery
11 seminiferous tubules

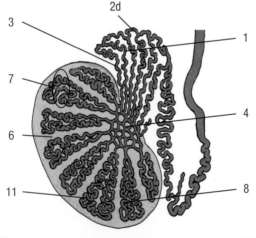

© A. L. Neill

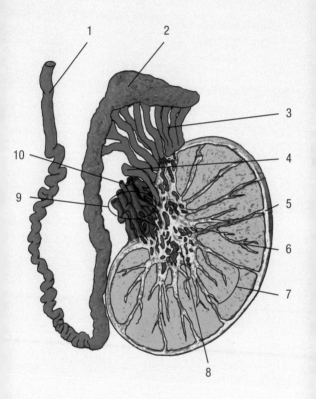

Testes - seminiferous tubules

Histology
LP H&E overview

1 tunica albuginia - capsule
2 tunica vasculosa
3 BV in the septum
4 septum
5 interstitial CT cells
6 seminferous tubule
7 interstitial cells of Leydig

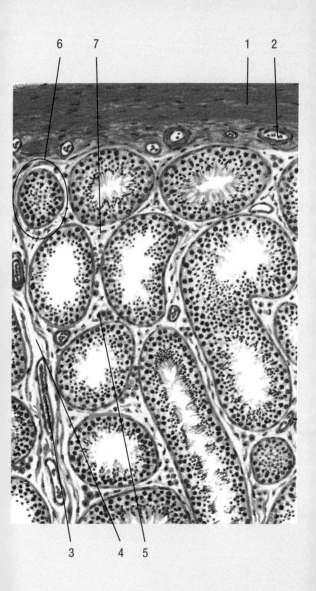

6   7   1   2

3   4   5

Testis
Examination (TE)

Palpation

A   examination of the testes & scrotum

B   examination of the spermatic cord

C   exmination of the shaft of the penis

Monthly self testicular examination (TSE) is recommended for boys/men > 14 yo. as testicular cancer is the commonest form of cancer in young males, although still very rare. When relaxed (to avoid the cremasteric reflex) - often after a bath and with warm hands examine both testes. Both should feel the same size, soft & rubbery with a separate body behind & superiorly, the epididymis. The spermatic cord is posterior and should be the only hard cord felt in this region. If any other lump is felt during this procedure - follow up is recommended.

1   shaft of the penis
2   frenulum (note this is a circumcised penis)
3   testis
4   epididymis
5   spermatic cord

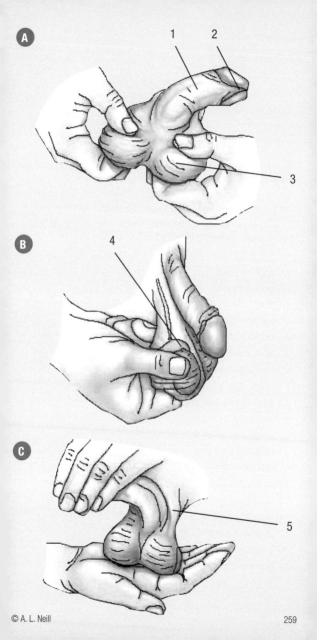

Urethra
Female

Macroscopic view

A   Coronal - cut through the bladder neck

B   Parasagittal - looking from the side

The bladder is a bag of multi-layered smooth muscle. It fills & empties from the base.   Abdominal P in the normal bladder has an equal effect on the bladder contents & the urethral opening. However with movement downwards of the bladder the urethral "sphincter" can move below the pelvic floor and hence abdominal P is only exerted on the body of the bladder and not equaled externally, putting excess P on the bladder opening and causing urinary incontinence.

1   muscular wall - extends down the neck = urethral sphincter

2   periurethral glands opening into the urethra

3   para-urethral glands opening into the urethra (Skene's glands, not shown)

4   external urethral meatus

5   labia minora

6   subcutaneous fat & T of the labia majora

7   round lig

8   deep fascia AKA Colles' fascia

9   bulbocavernosus m

10   vestibular gland lying in the superficial perineal compartment

11   urogenital diaphragm containing the deep transverse m

12   cavernous venous plexus

13   levator ani m

14   bladder neck

15   bladder musculature

16   anterior vaginal wall

17   internal urethral orifice - at the base of the trigone

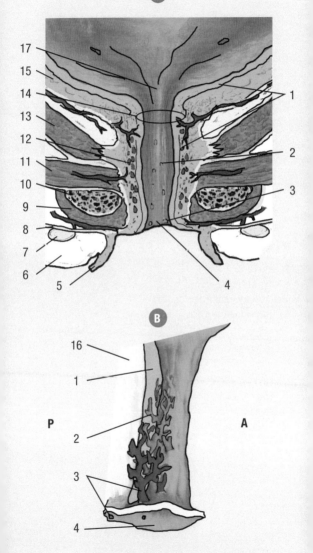

P   A

Uterus

Macroscopic Anterior frontal view
Coronal section

1. uterus -
     c = corp or body
     f = fundus
2. epoonphoron AKA parovarium (remanent of the mesonephric duct)
3. infundibulopelvic lig
4. plicae of the ampulla of the oviduct
5. fimbria
6. ovary
     A = corpus albicans
     f = follicle
     L = corpus luteum
7. ovarian lig
8. broad lig
9. uterine a & v
10. cut edge of the peritoneum
11. cardinal lig AKA Mackenrodt's lig
12. cervix
     e = externa os
     i = internal os
13. vaginal fornix
14. endocervical canal
15. vagina
16. mesosalpinx

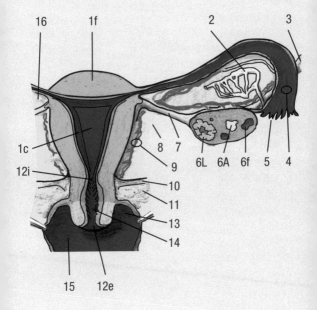

16   1f   2   3

1c

12i

8   7

6L   6A   6f   5   4

9

10

11

13

14

15   12e

Uterus
Cell Types

Endometrial glandular epithelial cell
Schema HP

The main cells lining the uterus in the secretory phase are the endometrial glandular epithelial cells. They are polarized elongated cells with mvs, glycogen & lipid stores & a specialized nuclear-cytoplasmic communication device the nucleolar channel system. The secretory granules increase with the growth of the endometrial wall, as do the lipofuscin containing vacuoles, which are present in aging cells.

1 cytoplasmic
     i = invagination
2 mv
3 secretory granule containing mucopolysaccharides
4 fibrils
     t = terminal web
5 mitochondria
6 GA
7 lipofuscin droplets
8 lipid droplets
9 nucleus
     m = nuclear membrane
     p = pore
10 ER
     S = smooth ER
     R = rough ER (ribosomes attached)
11 nucleolus
12 glycogen granules
13 nucleolar channel system

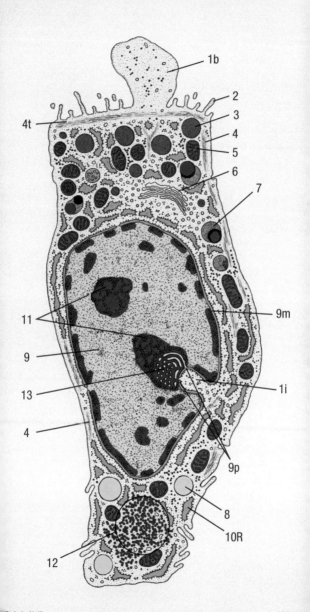

Uterus
Cell Types

Endometrial granulocytes
Schema HP

Large spherical granular cells are abundant in the stroma of the uterine lining - the endometrial granulocytes. It is thought their function may be to facilitate implantation & secretion of relaxin.

1   cytoplasmic
    b = blebs
    i = invagination
2   ribosomes
3   secretory granule
    p = protein/ enzymic
4   fibrils
5   mitochondria
6   GA
7   lipofuscin
8   lipid droplets
9   nucleus
    m = nuclear membrane
    p = pore
10 ER
    S = smooth ER
    R = rough ER (ribosomes attached)
11 nucleolus
12 glycogen granules
13 centromeres
    t = tubules

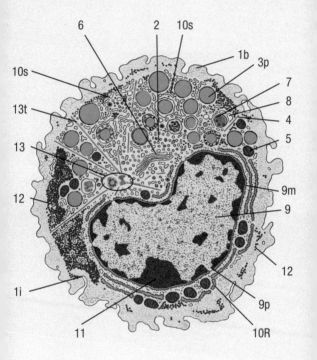

10s

6　　2　10s

　　　　　　　　　1b

　　　　　　3p

13t

13

12

1i

11

267

© A. L. Neill

7

8

4

5

9m

9

12

9p

10R

Uterine wall

Histology –

A *LP proliferative phase*

B *LP secretory phase*

C *LP menstral phase*

The uterine wall changes dramatically throughout the menstrual cycle, beginning with **the proliferative phase** where the mucosa builds up after its loss from menstruation; the glands and mucosa then become engorged with secretions under the influence of the CL – **the secretory phase** and finally 70-80% the mucosa is then sloughed off when a fertilization does not occur – **the menstral phase**.

1 endometrium – mucosa of the uterus
- b = basal layer – from which the new tissue will develop
- f = functional layer – layer which will provide nourishment for the implanted ovum
- r = residual layer – that remaining after menstrual bleeding

2 myometrium – muscle layer of the uterine wall

3 epithelial lining of the uterus
- a = absent or sloughed off

4 lamina propria

5 coiled arterioles

6 uterine glands
- b = blood filled & necrotic
- e = engorged & tortuous

7 smooth muscle layers in various planes, the uterus muscle is multilayered and highly vascular – flattens out and thins as the uterus swells with the engorged endometrium

8 a & v

9 sloughed off tissue – glandular & lamina propria

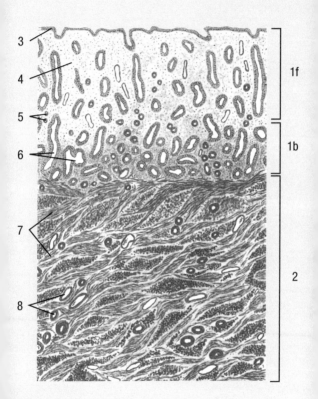

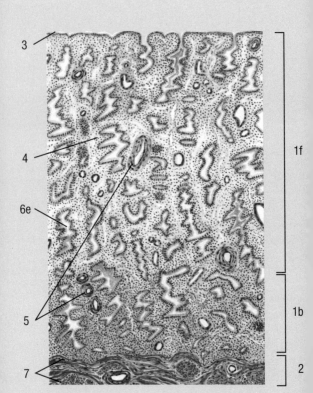

© A. L. Neil

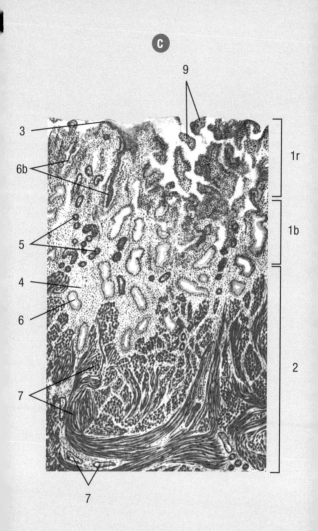

C

© A. L. Neill

Uterus
Blood Supply - Anastomoses

Schema

The BS of the uterus comes from branches on the internal iliac and is intimately related to that of the adjacent structures, such as the vaginal BVs from the hypogastric. The intimate relationship b/n the uterine and the ureter is important to note - particularly in procedures such as an hysterectomy.

1   uterus - fundus
2   ovarian tube
3   ampulla
4   ovarian a - br from the aorta
5   ovary
6   ureter
7   internal iliac a
      p = internal pudendal
      m = middle rectal
      u = uterine
      v = vaginal
8   perineal a
9   vestibule
10 cervix

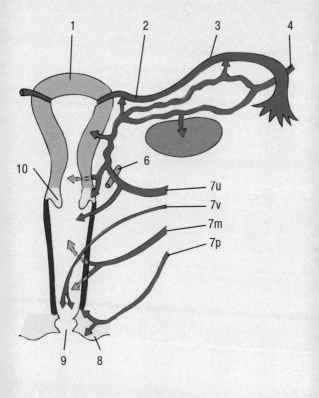

Uterus
Changes with age

1 new born - note is larger than that of the infant

2 infant about 3yo

3 13yo girl - at puberty 1/2 above & 1/2 below the isthmus line

4 adult - nulliparous

5 adult - multiparous

6 menopausal female - note there is a higher fibrous content of this organ   -

7 line of the isthmus & anterior peritoneal reflection note in the infant & menopausal uterus this line divides the uterus in to 2/3 cervix & 1/3 fundus

8 uterine cavity of the fundus

9 cervix - note elongates in the pregnant uterus

10 os AKA entrance of the cervix

     e = external os

     i = internal os

11 cervical mucous glands

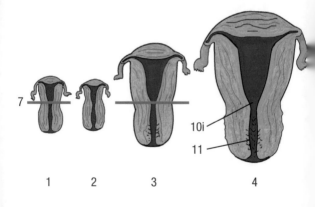

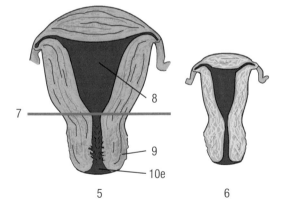

7 ——————

8

9

10e

5

6

Uterus

A   Growth in Pregnancy

B   Ligamentous support

The uterus increases with the development of the pregnancy.

It may be palpated abdominally when it rises above the pelvic brim, >12 weeks gestation, at which time the foetal heart beat may be detected.   The uterus continues to increase in size by 2 fingerbreadths for the next 8 weeks after which it grows at half that rate, until delivery.

Quickening - or movement of the foetus occurs at ~approximately 18 weeks.

1   vulva + perineum - shows signs of damage &repair after pregnancy

2   PS - softens in later pregnancy under hormonal influence to allow for the passage of the foetal head

3   stria gravidarum - initially bright red or purple they settle to become white lines indicating weakened skin with surface collagen

4   umbilicus

5   costal margin

6   xiphisternum

7   areola & nipple - which often become irreversibly pigmented with pregnancy

8   breast tissue - which grows & swells with the pregnancy as the glands develop & become engorged with milk - after lactation the glands devolve and the T loses a lot of its firmness

9   weeks of pregnancy - note in the last 2 weeks the uterus will drop ready for delivery

10 ovarian lig

11 round lig

12 uterosacral lig

13 cardinal lig

14 vaginal wall

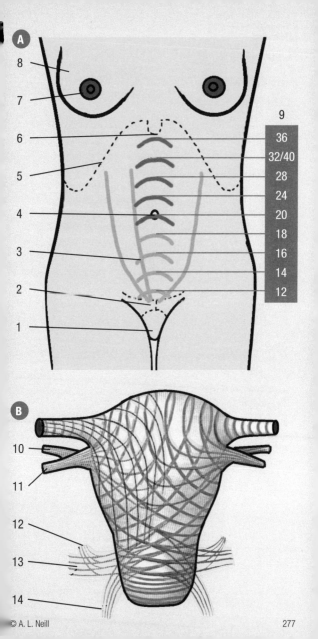

Uterine "Malposition" Anteversion, Retroversion/Retroflexion & Incarceration

Schema

The normal uterus moves around freely in the pelvic cavity, via a central pivot. Anteversion is considered the normal position but Retroversion is a normal anomaly in 20% of females. Alone retroversion is not normally associated with pelvic pain or dysmenorrhea and does not need correction, however fixed retroversion may be associated with pathology such as: interference in defecation/urination and may lead to incarceration or trapping of the uterus behind the sacral promontory. The terms flexion & version are used interchangeably, however it may be considered that flexion is slightly more severe.

1 anteversion
2 retroversion - normal in 20% of females
    i = primary
    ii = secondary
    iii = tertiary
3 retroflexion (note also 2)
4 pivot of rotation & uterine movement
5 p = pubis
    s = sacrum
6 colon - altered contour with severe or fixed retroversion

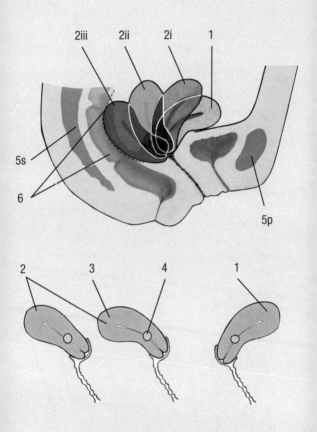

© A. L. Neill

Uterus
Prolapse

A Primary Prolapse - slight descent
B Secondary Prolapse - cervix at the introitus (entrance)
C Tertiary Prolapse - complete displacement - irreversible
D Tertiary Prolapse - surface appearance

The uterus may be displaced from its primary position due to internal abdominal pressure, weakening of its supportive ligaments, diminishing size of the uterus &/or laxity of the vaginal walls. Multiparous women are more likely to have this condition particularly if they have multiple births & are obese. Once past the entrance an hysterectomy is inevitable, after which the vaginal walls may be need to be supported and attached to pelvic structures.

1 **Pubis**
2 **bladder**
3 **urethra - note the change in direction with increasing prolapse**
4 **anus**
5 **perineal body - compromised with the prolapse**
6 **clitoris - moved closer to the Pubis on prolapse**

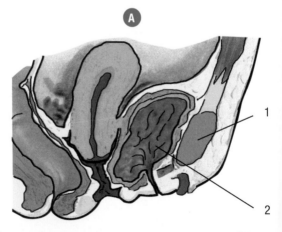

A

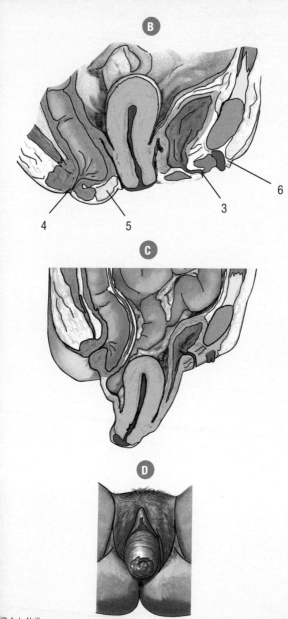

Uterine Prolapse + Enterocele + Rectocele

Macroscopic - Sagittal view

When there is a shift in position of any of the pelvic organs it may result in other related shifts and functional compromises. The same ligament support system of the uterus also supports other organs in the area.

1 Pubis
2 bladder
3 urethra
4 anus
5 perineal body stretched with the enterocele
6 clitoris - moved closer to the Pubis on prolapse
7 cystocele (stage 1)
8 uterine prolapse (2-3rd degree)
9 enterocele AKA intestinal prolapse
10 rectocele AKA rectal prolapse

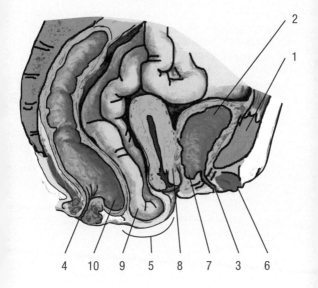

4   10   9   5   8   7   3   6

Vaginal wall

Histology –

A   LP overview H&E

B   HP epithelial lining interfollicular phase Mancini's iodine technique

C   HP epithelial lining follicular phase

The vaginal wall uterine changes minimally throughout the menstrual cycle. Mainly the epithelial lining is affected, proliferating & accumulating glycogen in the follicular stage under oestrogen influence until it is maximal around ovulation. The surface cells are then shed & the bacterial flora in the lumen metabolize the sugar, forming acid, which protects the vagina from pathogenic MOs. Iodine is used to detect the amount of starch in the vaginal wall.

1   BVs in the mucosa

2   CT papilla

3   stratified squamous epithelium
    s = surface layers dead dying filled with glycogen
    d = deep layers w/o glycogen

4   CT under the epithelium AKA Lamina propria

5   adventitia

6   smooth muscle bands
    L = longitudinal
    T = transverse

7   lymphoid T

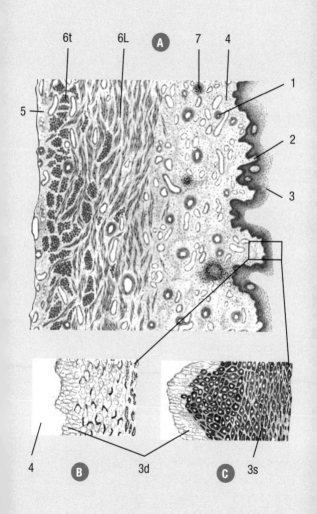

Vagina
Examination

A   *digital examination - vulva removed*
B   *specular examination*
C   *cervical examination - cytology sampling, punch biopsy
     & cone biopsy*
D   *cervical sites - taken for cytology*
E   *Pap smear showing mild dysplasia*
F   *colposcopic examination*

The vagina is a fibromuscular tube connecting the outside to the uterus, used to introduce the sperm to the egg & the passage of the birth (AKA birth canal). It is flat with horizontal folds (rugae) & enormous elasticity. When opened the uterine cervix can be examined, & its surface sampled.

Inspect the vulval area, then examine the vagina is digitally & use this to assess any adnexal masses, the size /shape of the uterus. Using the speculum visualize & sample the cervix.

Results may show a number of changes in the cytology, leading to further examination with the colposcope (11).

1   internal digits - examining the vaginal wall integrity
2   "duck" speculum
3   vaginal lumen
4   sampling from the cervico-vaginal fornices (corners)
5   sampling from the cervix - external os
6   sampling from the cervix - surface
7   superficial cells
8   intermediate cells
9   endocervical cells - (from inside the external os)
10 cells with metaplastic changes
11 colposcope
12 direct light source

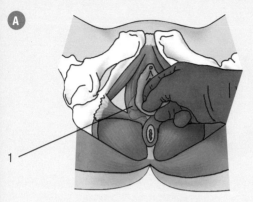

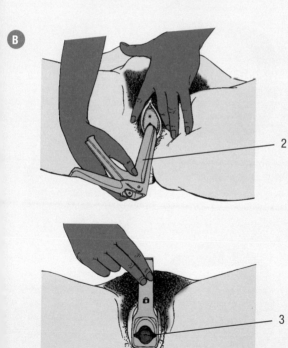

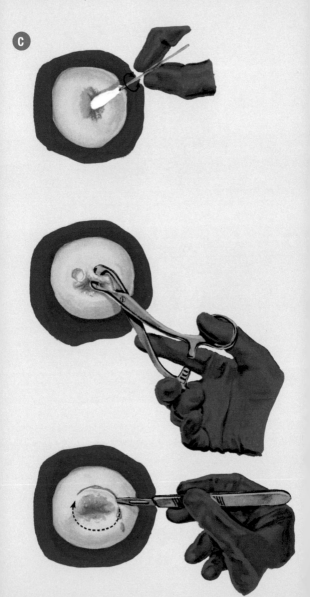

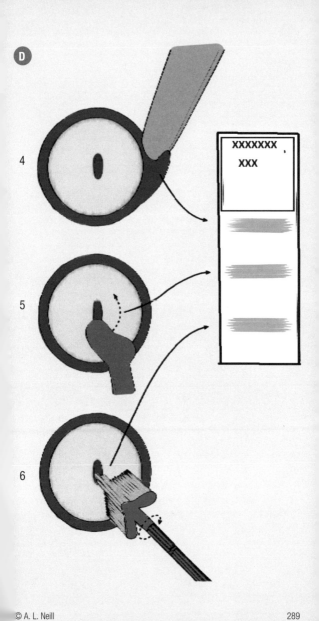

XXXXXXX

XXX

4

5

6

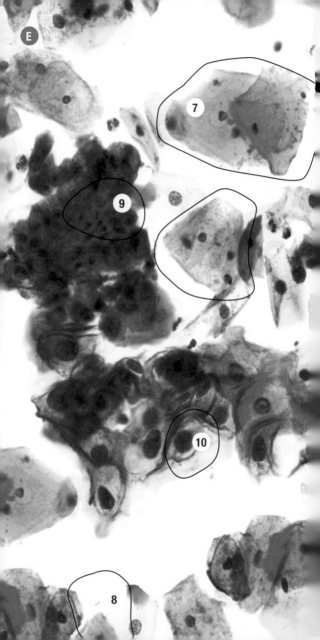

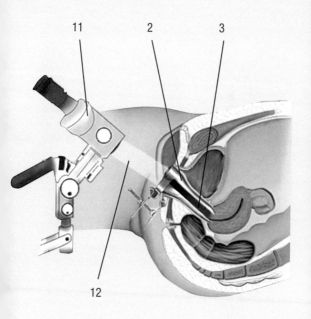

11

2   3

12

Vulva

Macroscopic view

*Inferior looking up into the Vulva, Vestibule & Vagina - open
Diagram of the outer "closed area"*

The vulva is the exposed external female genitalia. The space
between the 2 labia minora is the vestibule, where the delicate
contents are further protected. There is considerable variation in the
size, colour & shape of the normal range of these components.

1 vulva - space b/n the inner thighs - external female genitalia
2 pudendal cleft space b/n the labia majora
3 vestibule space and contents b/n the labia minora AKA
   interlabial sulci
4 mons pubis - non gender specific name AKA mons veneris
   (mound of love) specifically female
5 commissure - bands of connecting tissue joining each side
       a = anterior
       p= posterior
6 clitoris
       g = glans of the clitoris (equivalent to the glans of
           the penis)
       h = hood of = prepuce of the clitoris (equivalent of
           the foreskin if the penis)
7 skene's glands - these are activated in sexual excitement
   (equivalent of male ejaculation)
8 labia
       a = majoris (large outer lips)
       i = minoris (smaller inner lips - although these may be
           larger and protrude outside of the outer lips
9 fossa naviculatis
10 anus
11 perineum - raphe of the area AKA perineal body
12 vaginal introitus - note the internal horizontal folds or rugae
    of the vagina
13 openings of the Bartholin's gland AKA greater vestibular
    glands (equivalent to the bulbourethral glands of the penis)
    lubricate the vagina when stimulated
14 carunculae myrtiformes (remnants of the perforated hymen)
15 external urethral meatus

© A. L. Neill

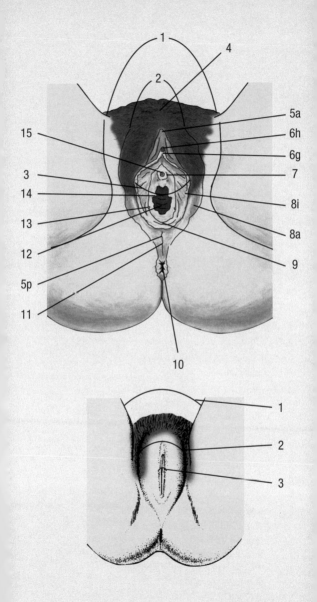

Vulva
Innervation

Macroscopic Inferior view - female
A - surface projection
B - deep dissection

The vulva has a similar innervation to that of the penis and scrotum, both are mainly supplied by the Pudendal N (S234). Additional sensory supply comes from the surrounding cutaneous Ns.

The Pudendal N is a mixed N palpable at its exit near the ischeal tuberosity. It innervates the muscles of the pelvic floor and the external anal sphincter, as well as the skin of the vulva and scrotum. It can be palpated in the female via the vagina, making a local block of this N possible.

This will cause the relaxation of all the muscles in the area and anaesthesia of the vulval area, and as such is often used in childbirth (shaded in blue).

The posterior femoral cutaneous N supplies the skin of the inner thigh and the back of the leg.

1   mons pubis
2   ilioinguinal N - ant labial branch
3   subcutaneous fat of the inner thigh
4   adductor muscles
5   posterior femoral cutaneous N (S1-2)
      g = gluteal branch (cluneal N)
      p = perineal branch
      t = branches to thigh and leg
6   gluteal muscles
7   sacrotuberous lig
8   perforating cutaneous N
9   anus
10 perineal body (PB)
11 pudendal N - muscular & cutaneous supply of the area
      c = dorsal N to the clitoris
      i = inf. haemorrhoidal N (AKA inf. rectal N)
      p = perineal N (d = deep branch)
      L = posterior labial
12 ischeal tuberosity

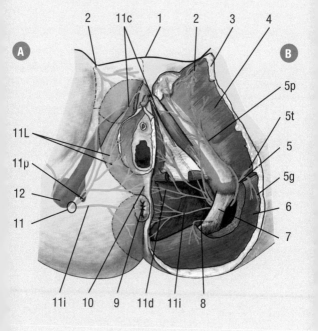

Vulva
Lacerations & Tears

Macroscopic view

A   first degree perineal laceration

B   second degree perineal laceration + clitoral tear

C   third degree laceration + labial tear

D   high vaginal laceration involving the cervix

In cases of sexual assault or misadventure the vulva may suffer several injuries. These are described as first, second & third degree along with ny accompanying injuries which are to be listed separately.

1   clitoris
2   urethra meatus
3   hymen - remnants
4   vaginal introitus
5   labia
      a = major
      l = minor
6   external anal sphincter
7   perneal body
8   cervix

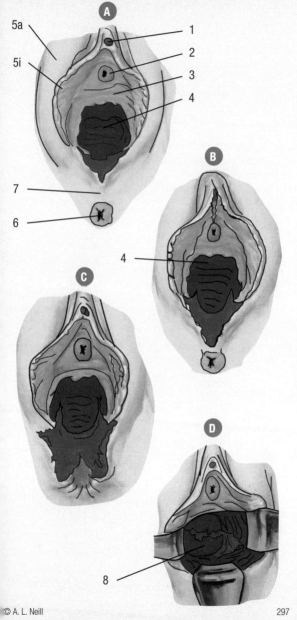

Vulva
Innervation
Pudendal Nerve
Examination & Block

Macroscopic   Inferior view - female

The external genitalia is innervated by the pudendal N, (S2-4). Hence the vulva can be anaesthetized by blocking this nerve, which can be found by pressing on the internal vaginal surface for the ischeal tuberosity and injecting 2 fingers further medially.

1   ischeal tuberosity
2   ischeal spine

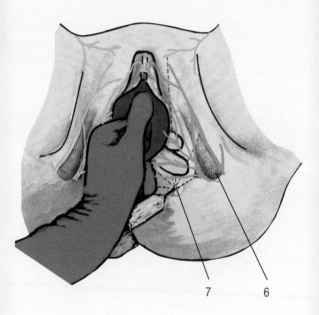

7   6

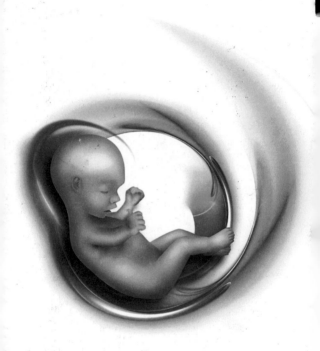